Thank you for bumy book of "Brain specifically designe conversation and give the memory a good workout.

Please look at each picture which is a zoomed in close-up of a familiar object. Try and work out what the object is. Some are quite easy and others not quite so easy.

Then turn to the next page to see if you got it right.

Giving the brain a workout is good for fun, confidence and returns the joy of remembering and achieving.

Good Luck

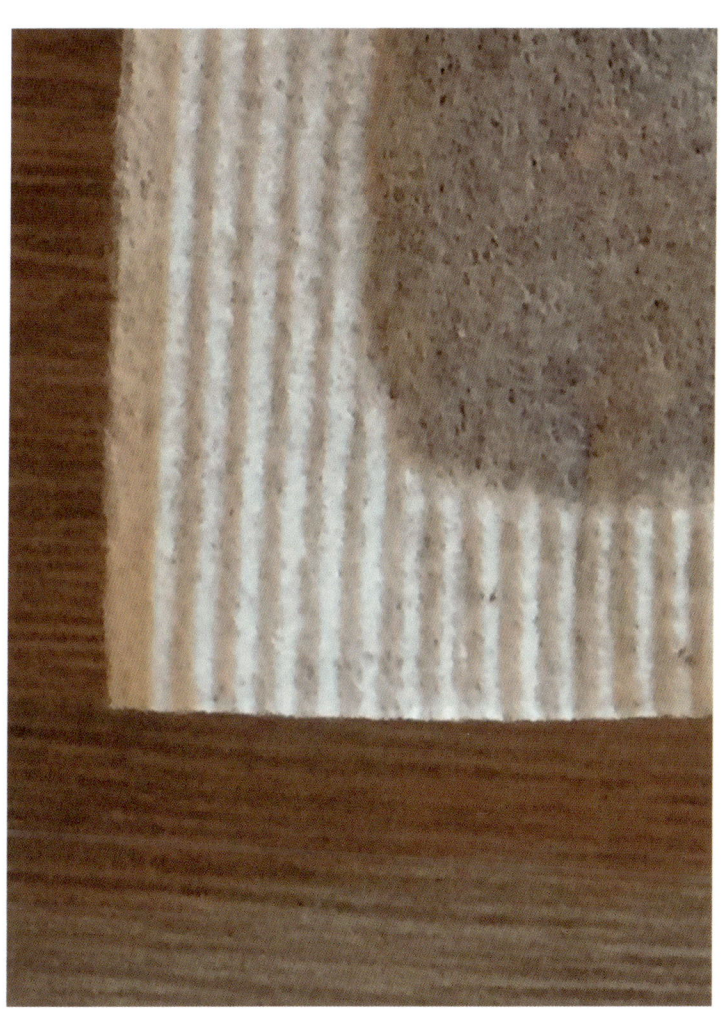

What is this?

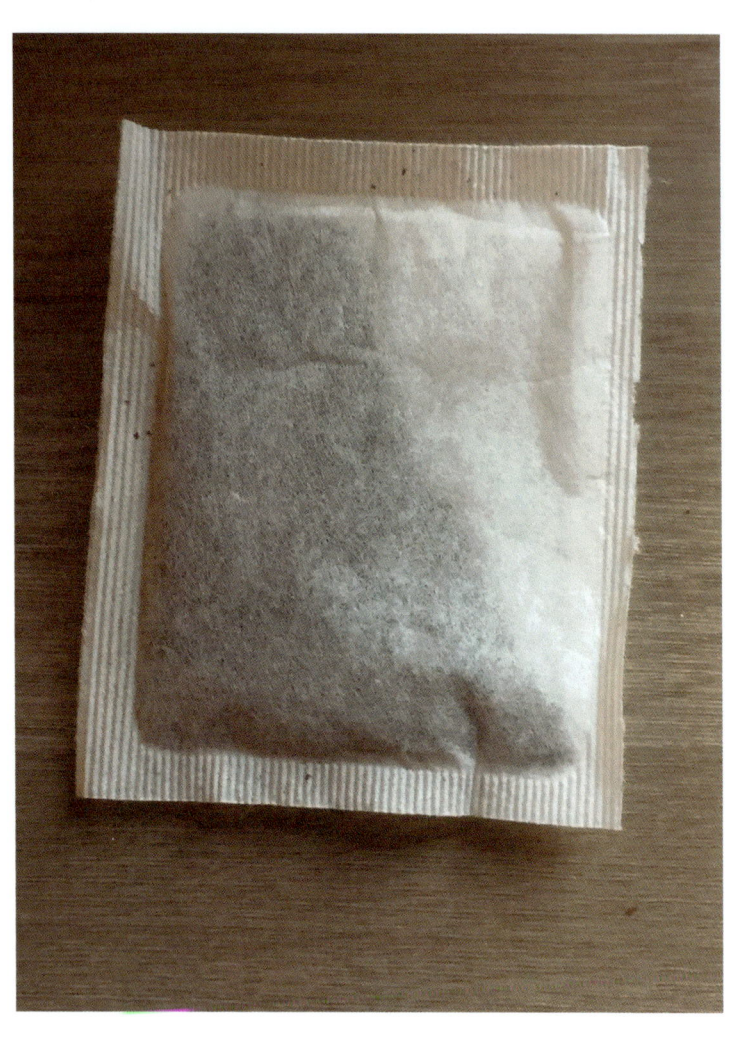

Tea Bag

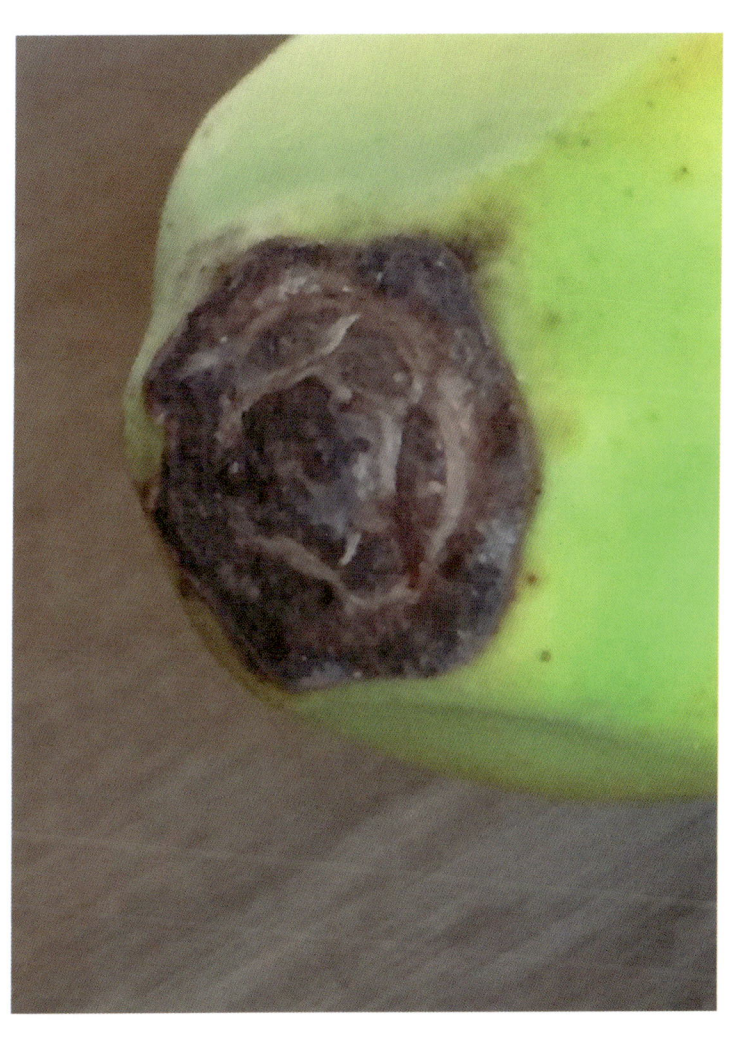

What is this?

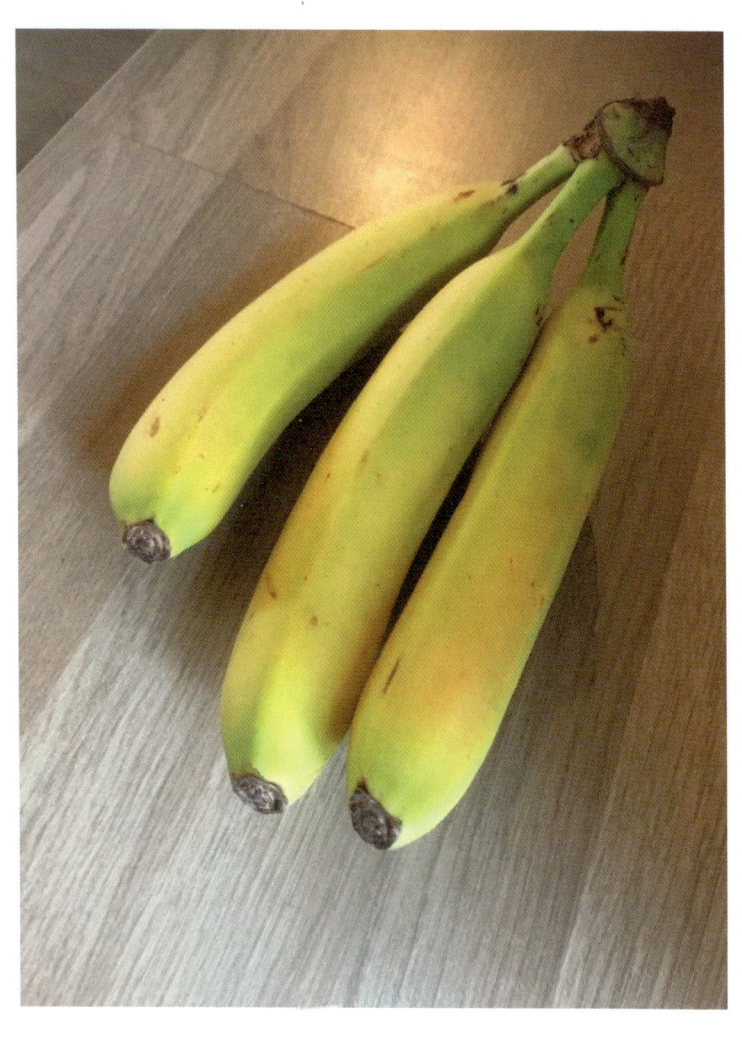

Banana.

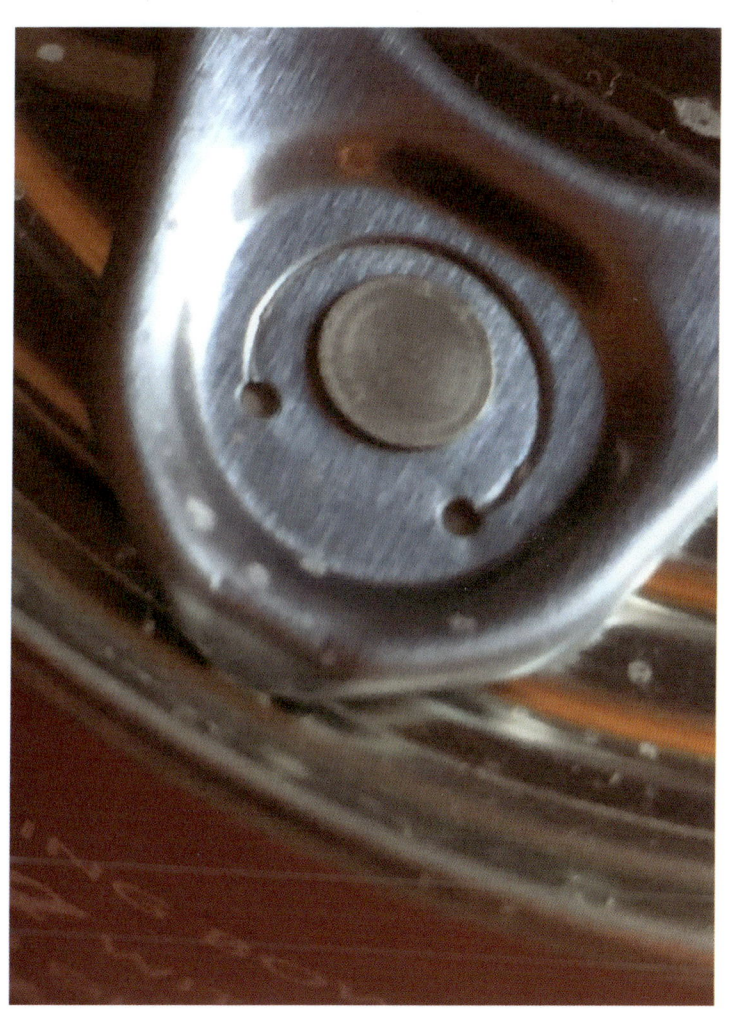

What is this?

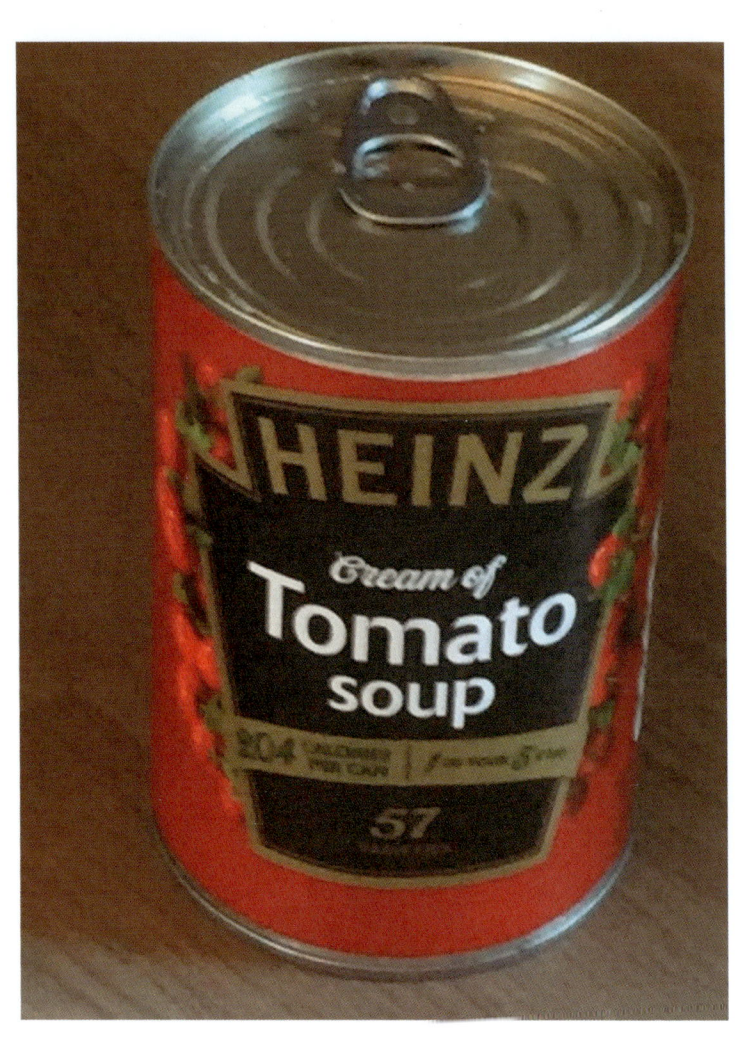

A tin.

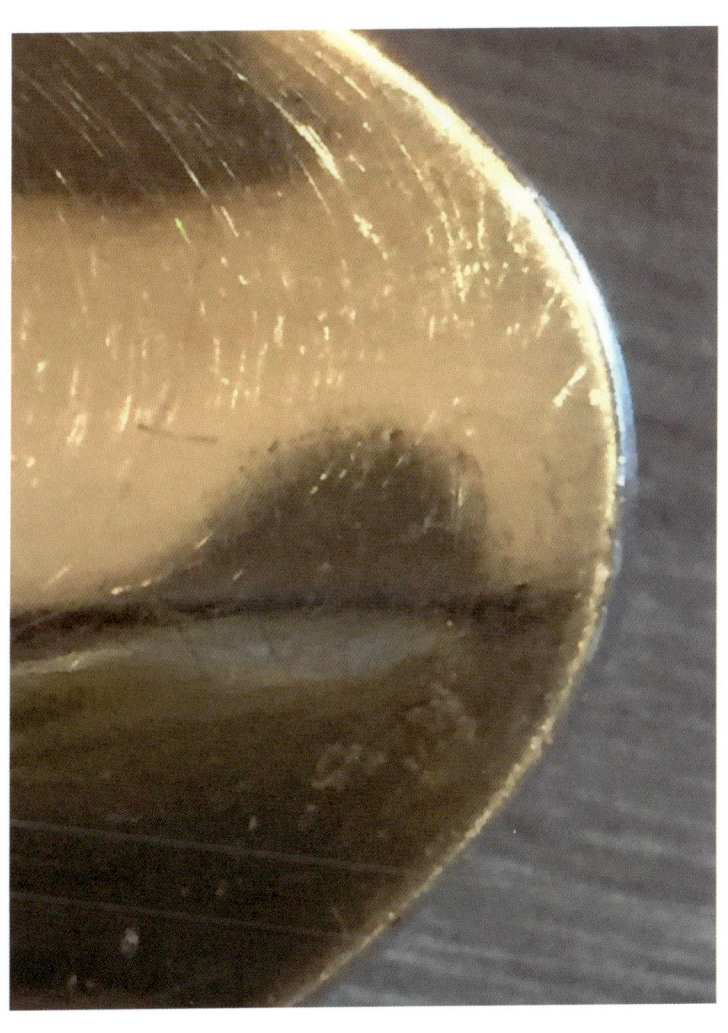

What could this be?

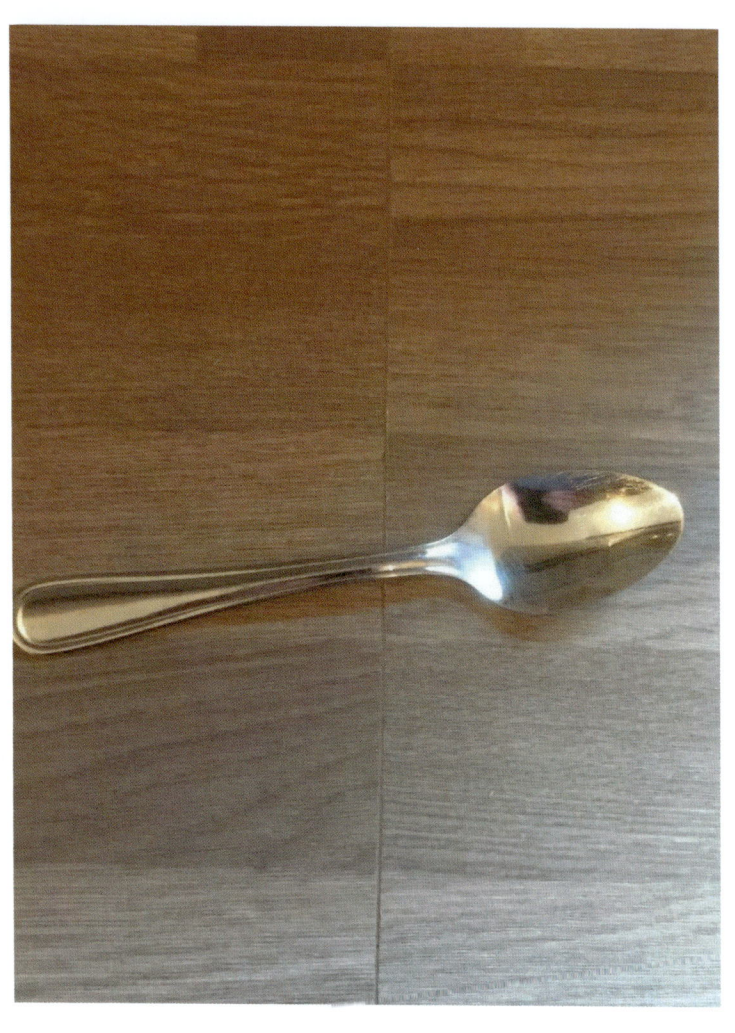

A spoon

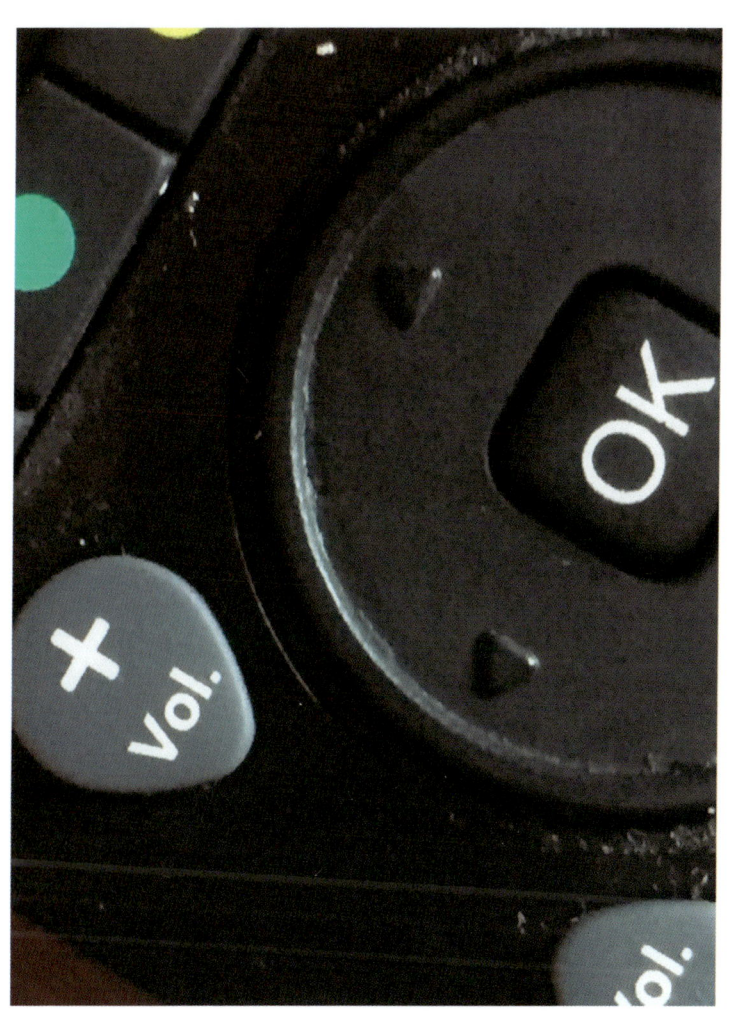

What is this?

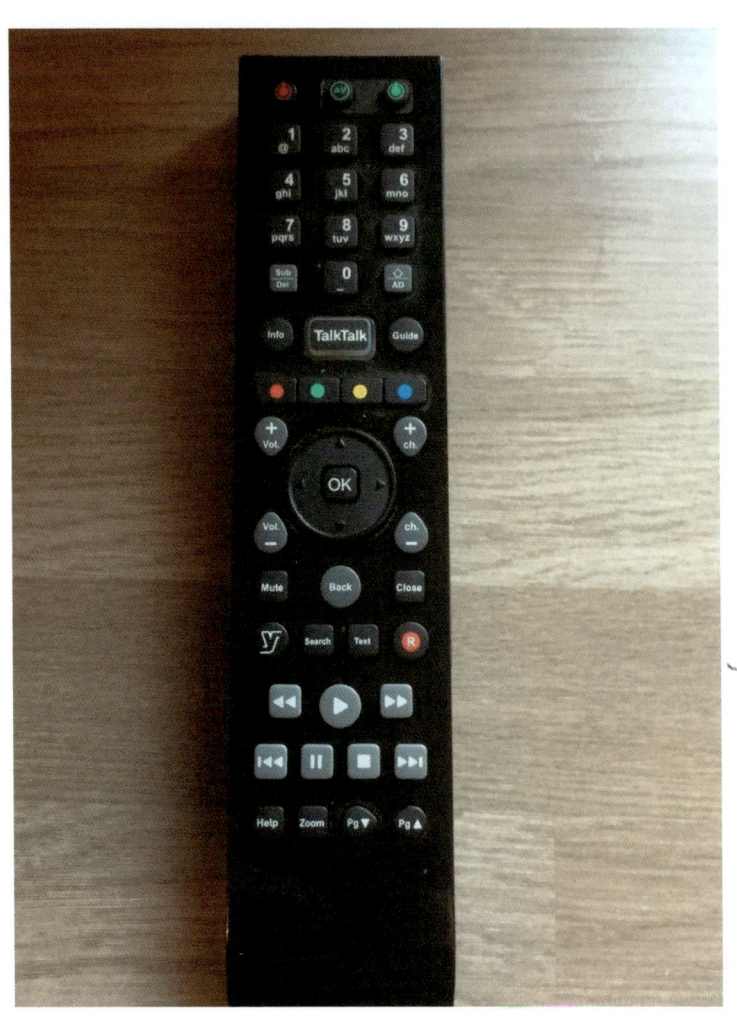

Remote Control

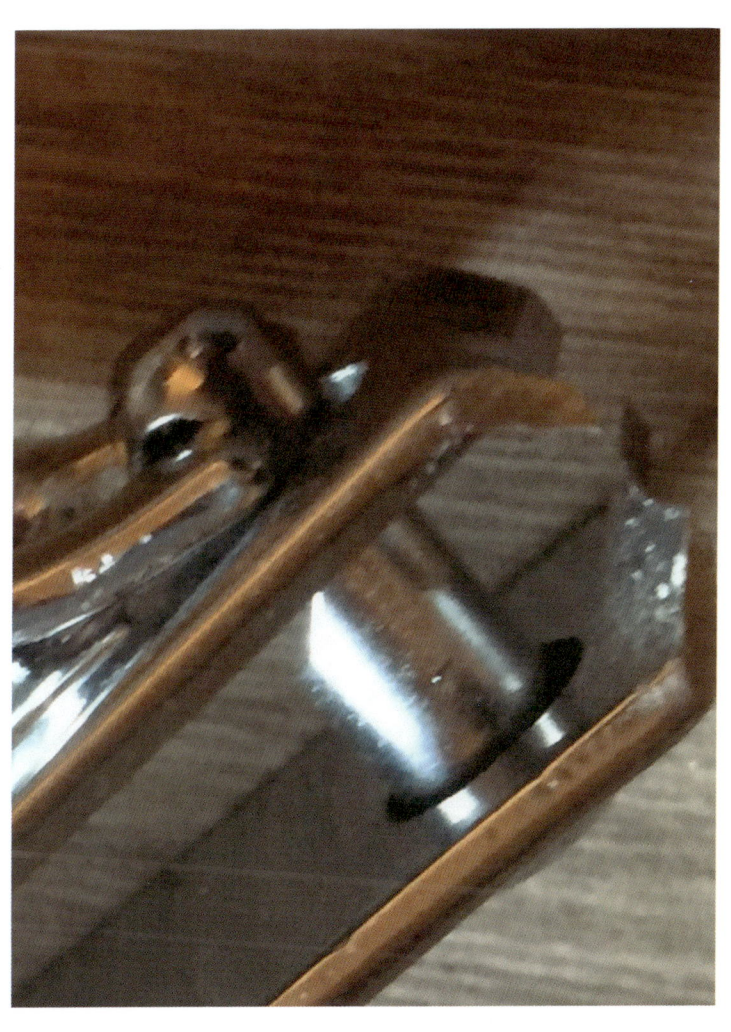

What might this be?

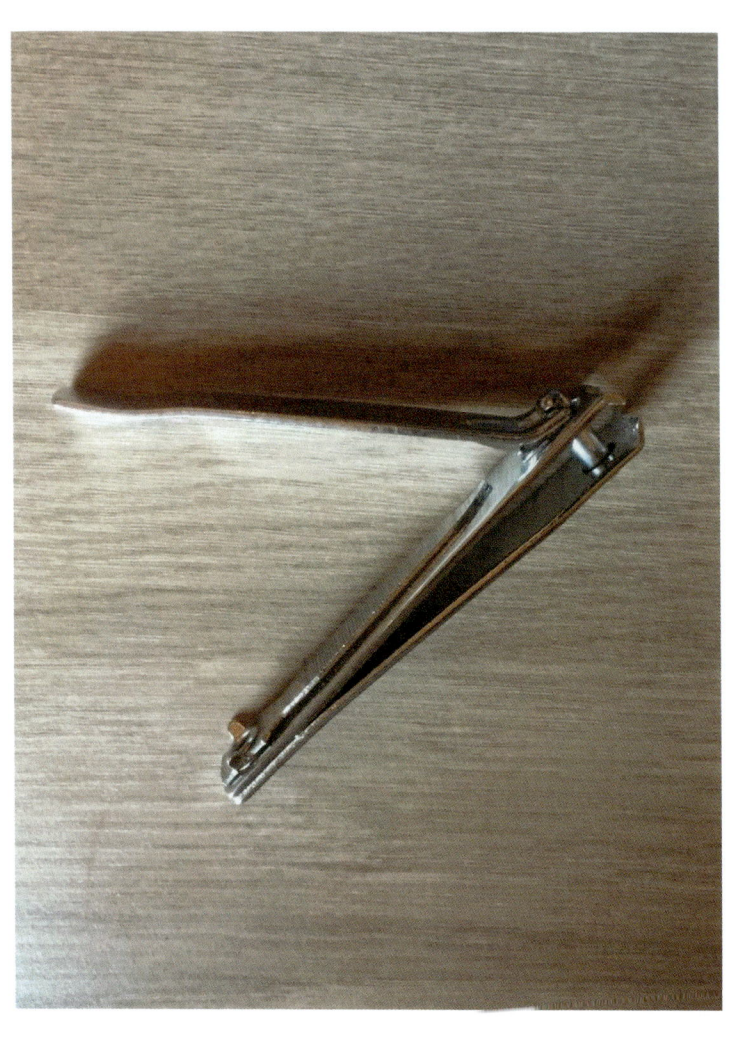

Nail Clippers

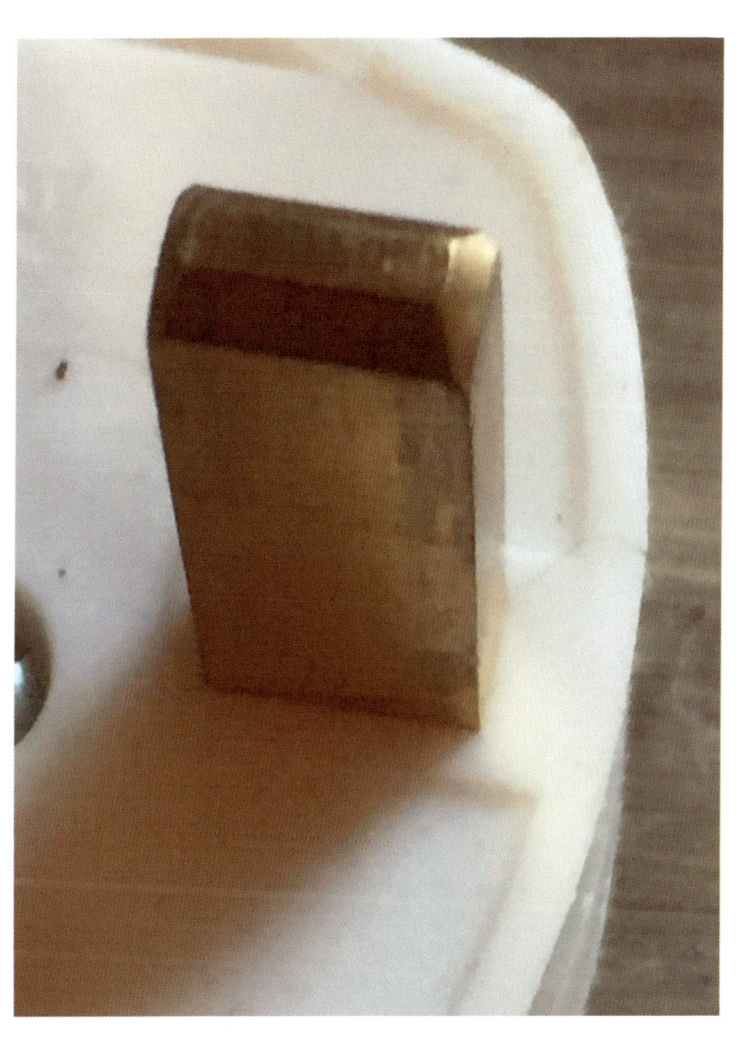

What is this?

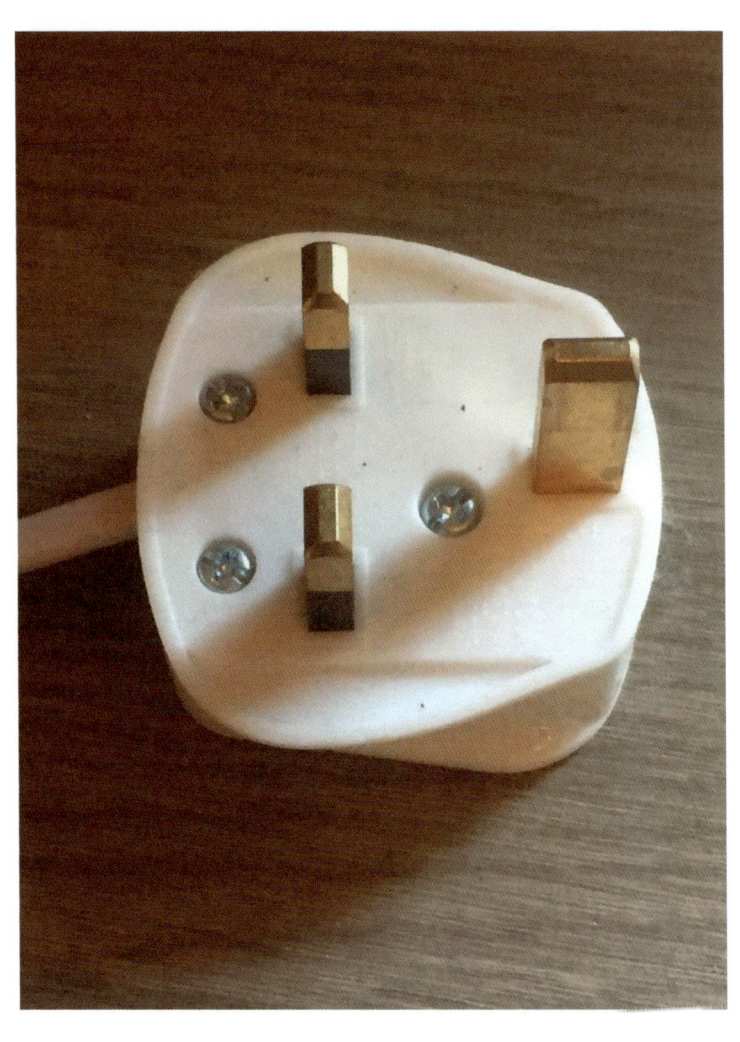

Electric Plug

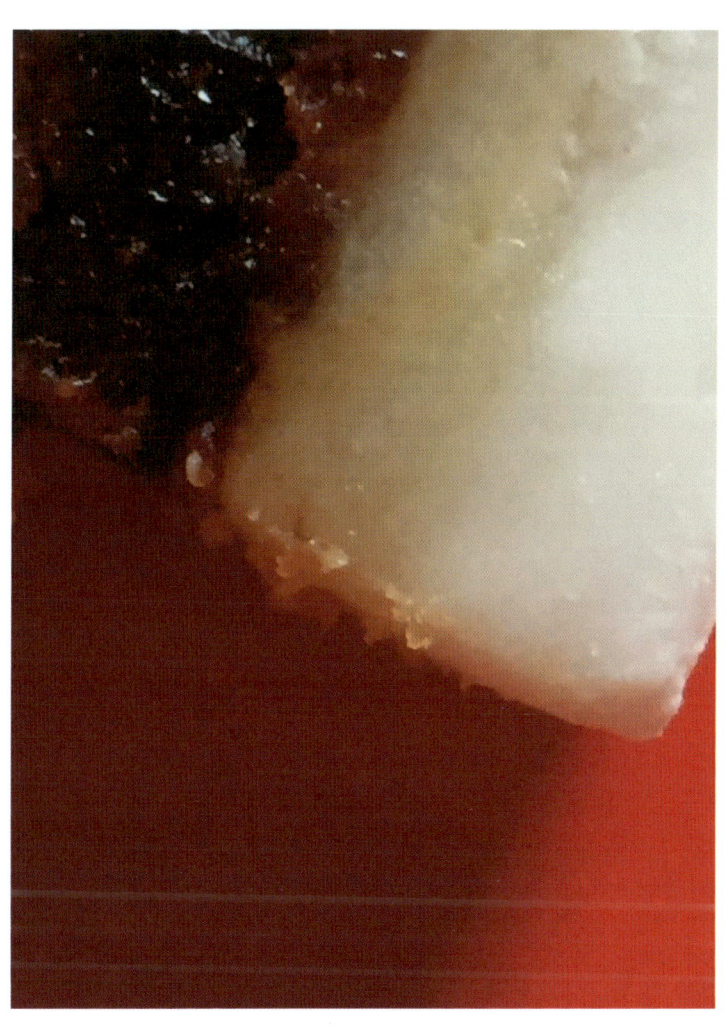

What might this be?

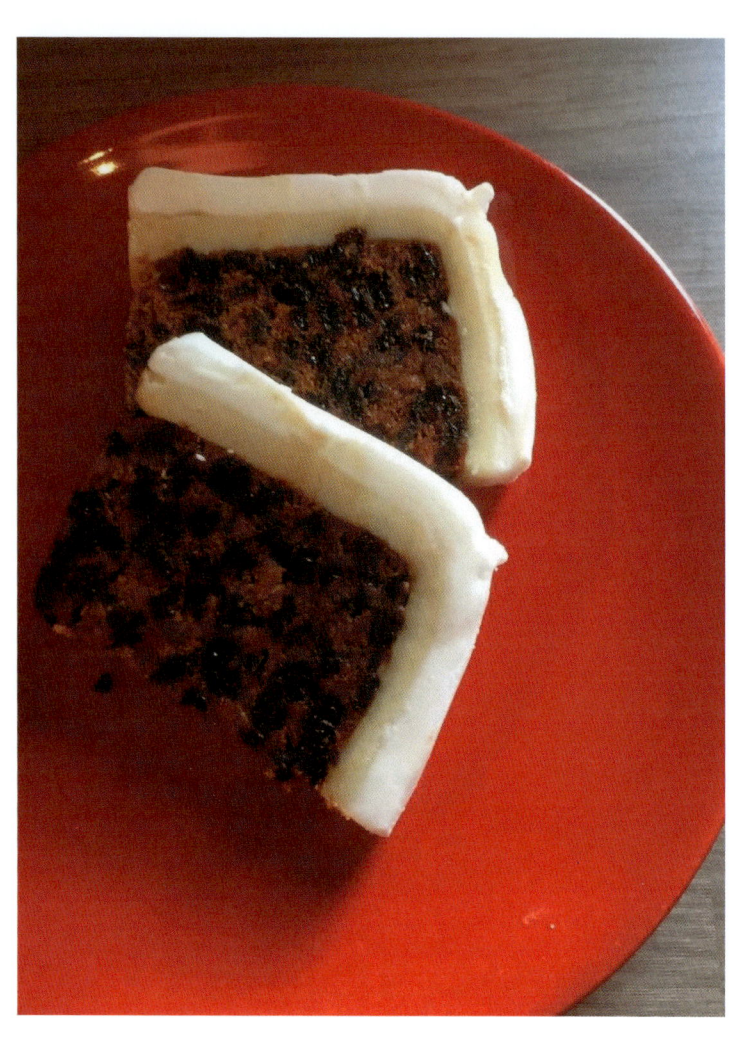

Fruit Cake

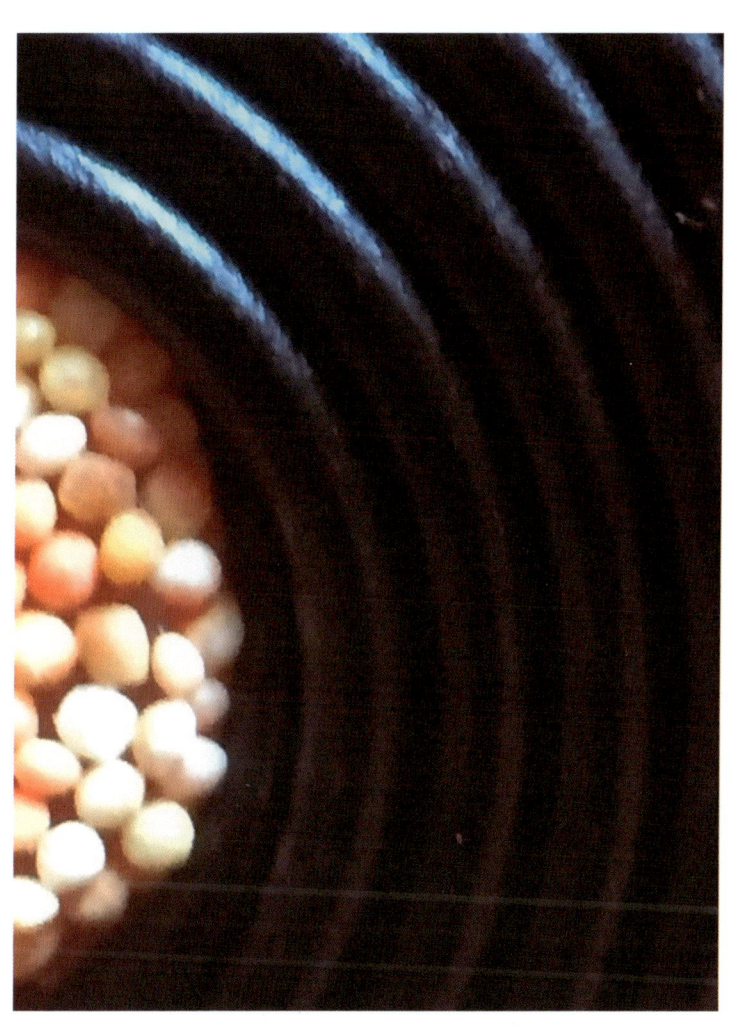

What's this?

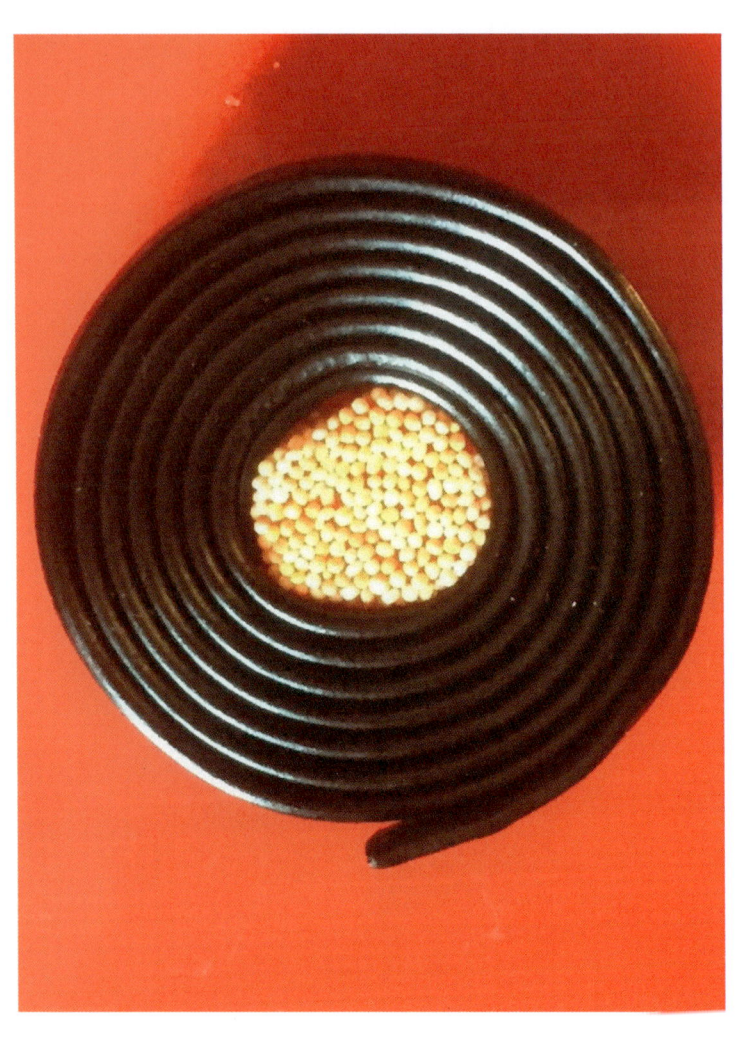

Liquorice

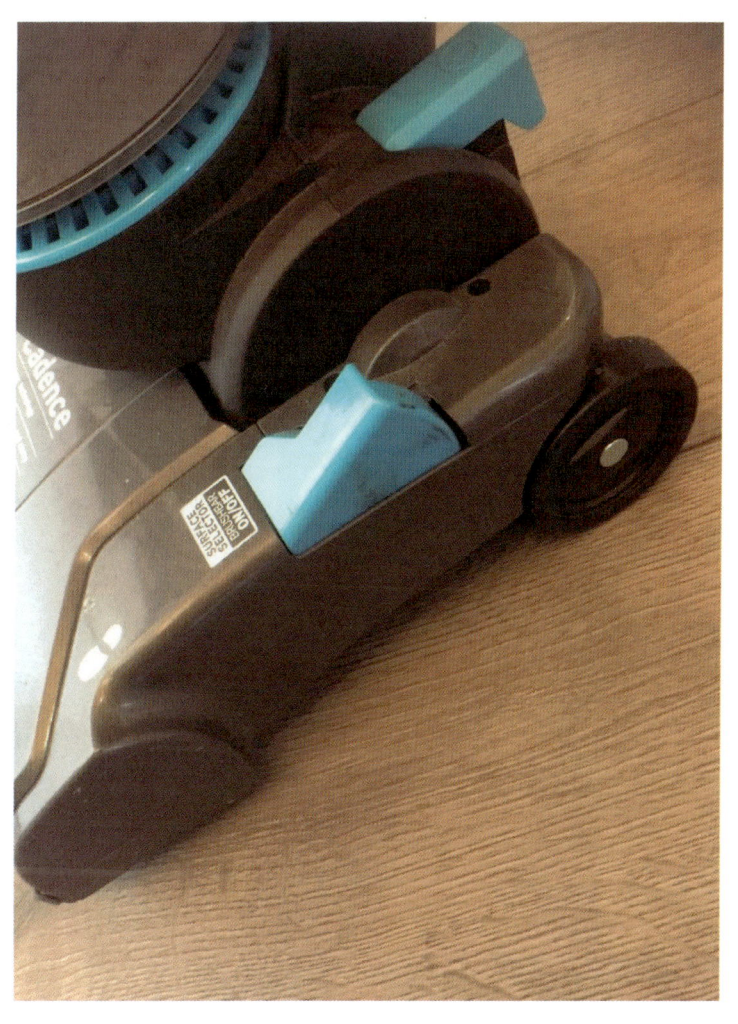

Do you recognise this?

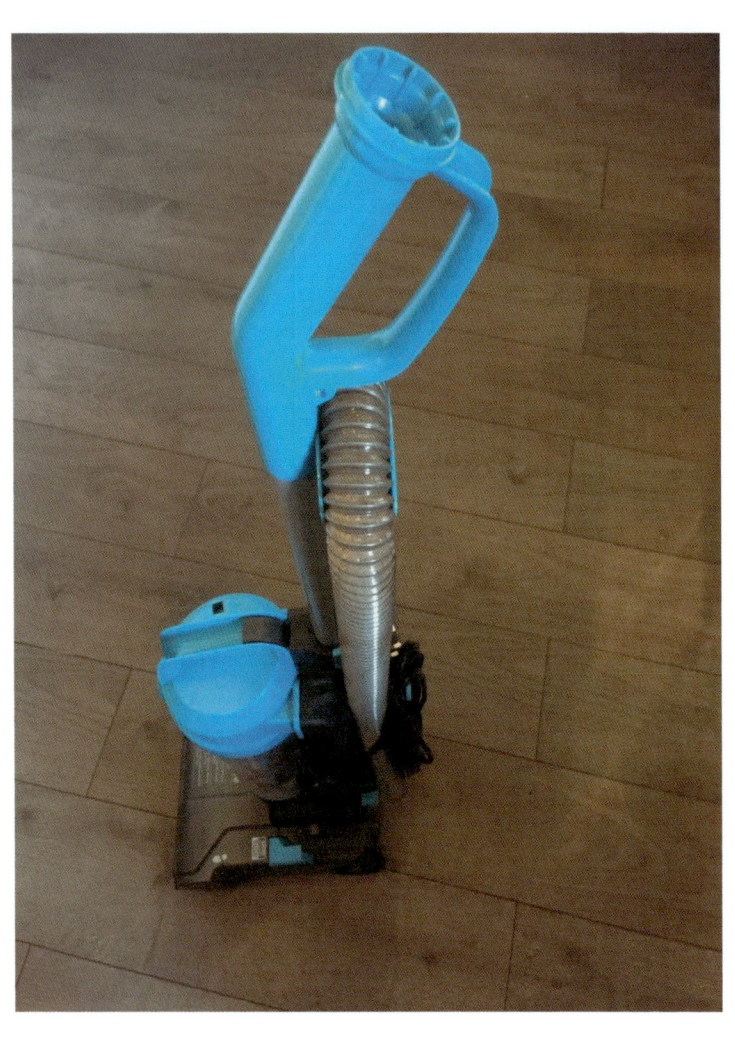

Hoover

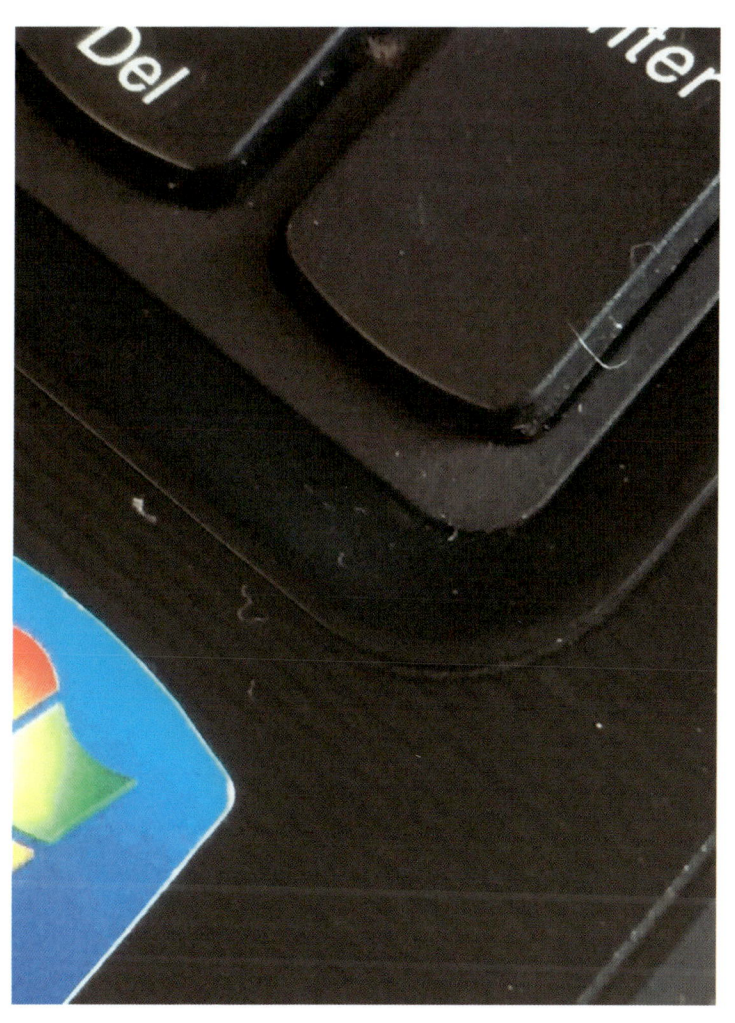

What is this part of?

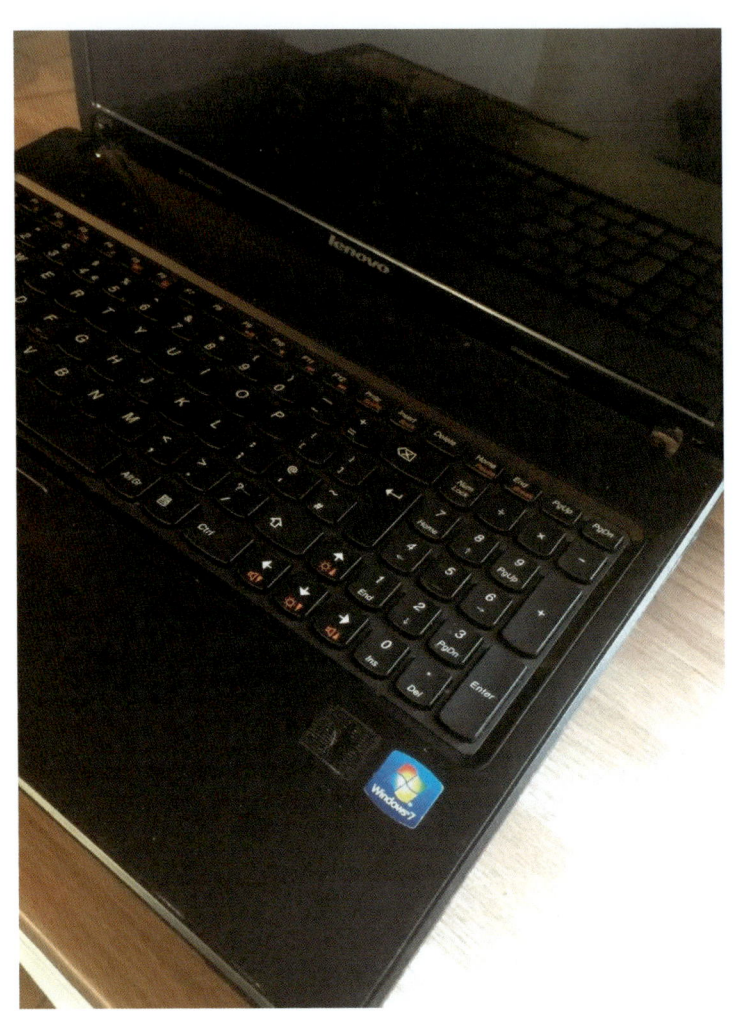

Laptop Computer

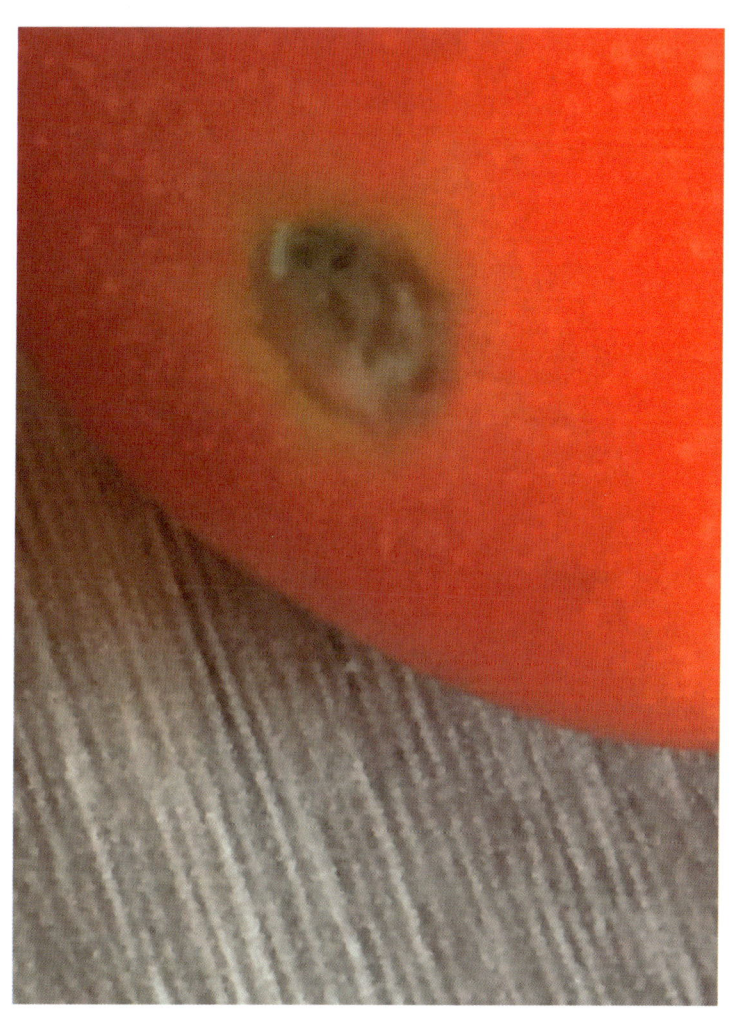

What food?

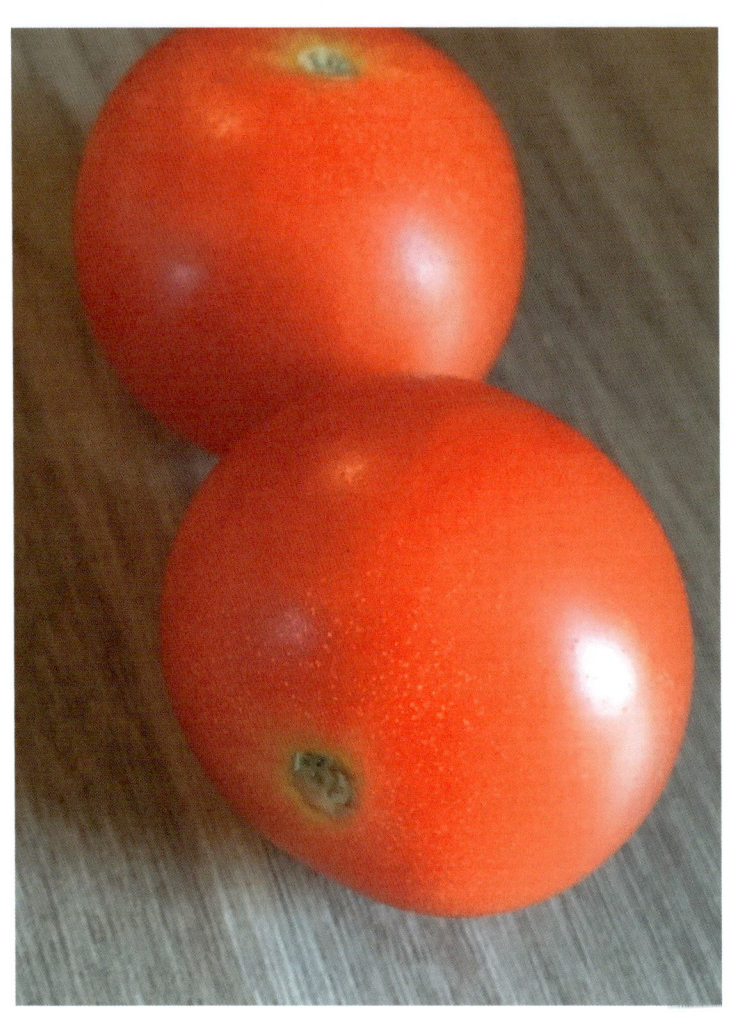

Tomato.

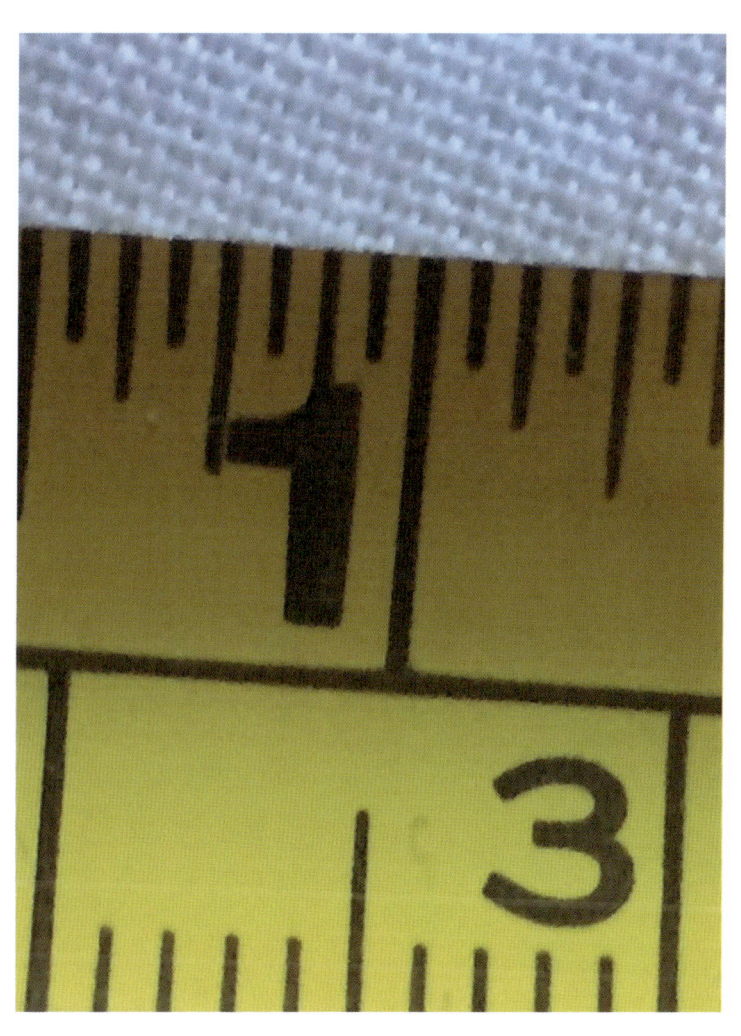

What is this?

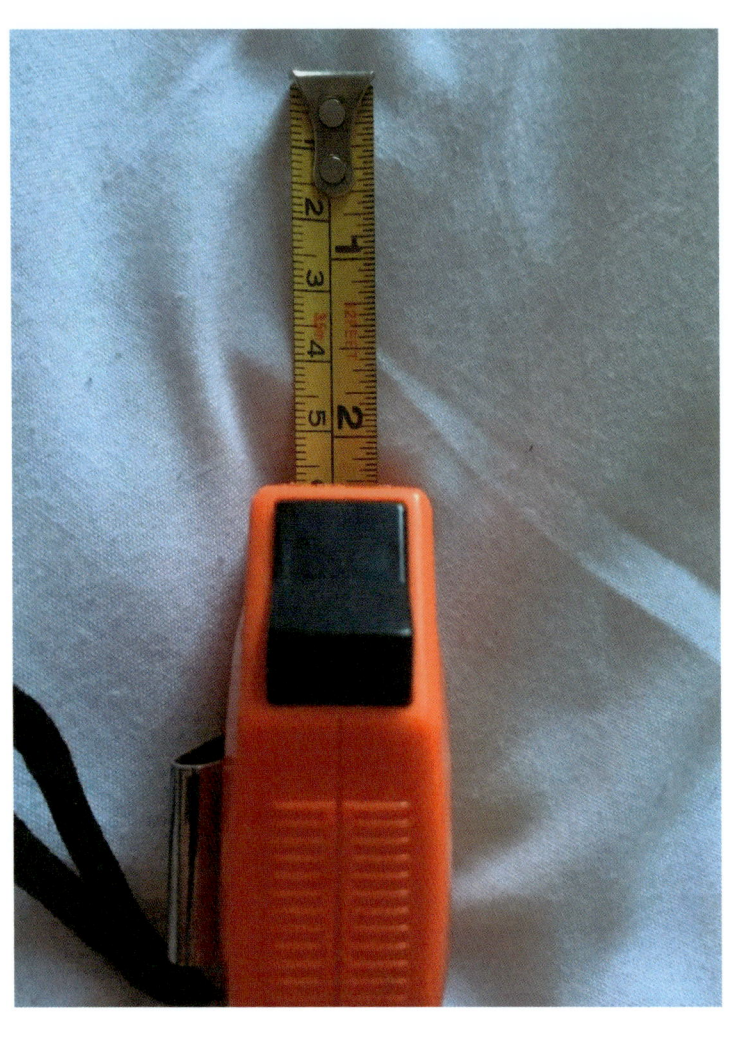

Tape measure.

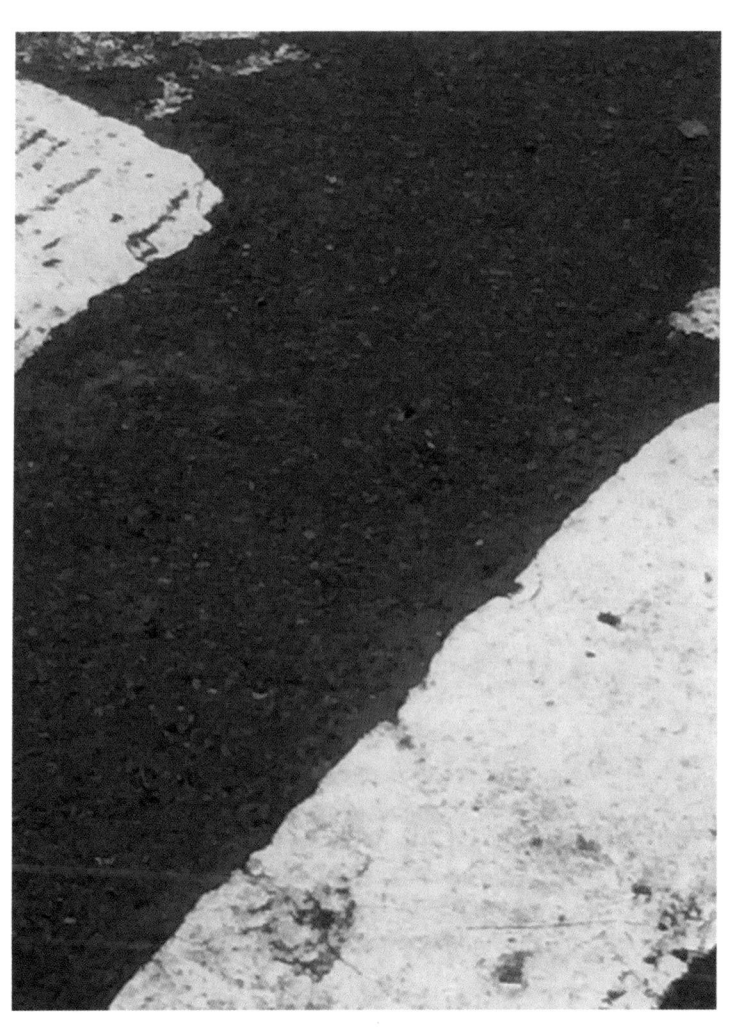

What are these?

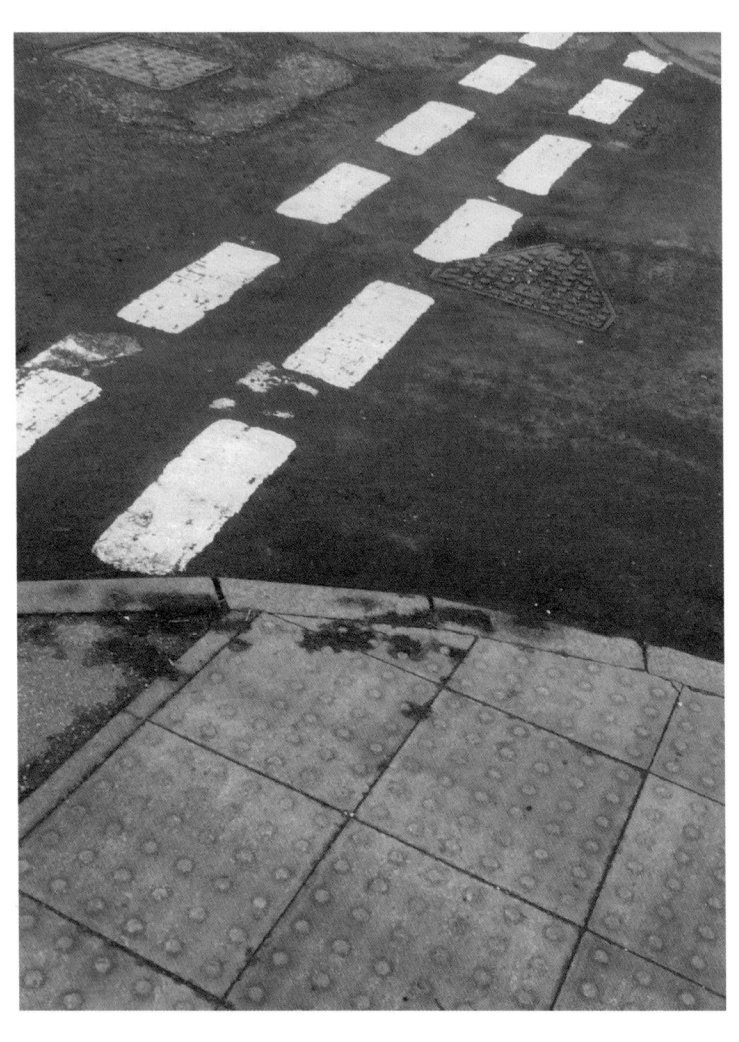

Road Markings

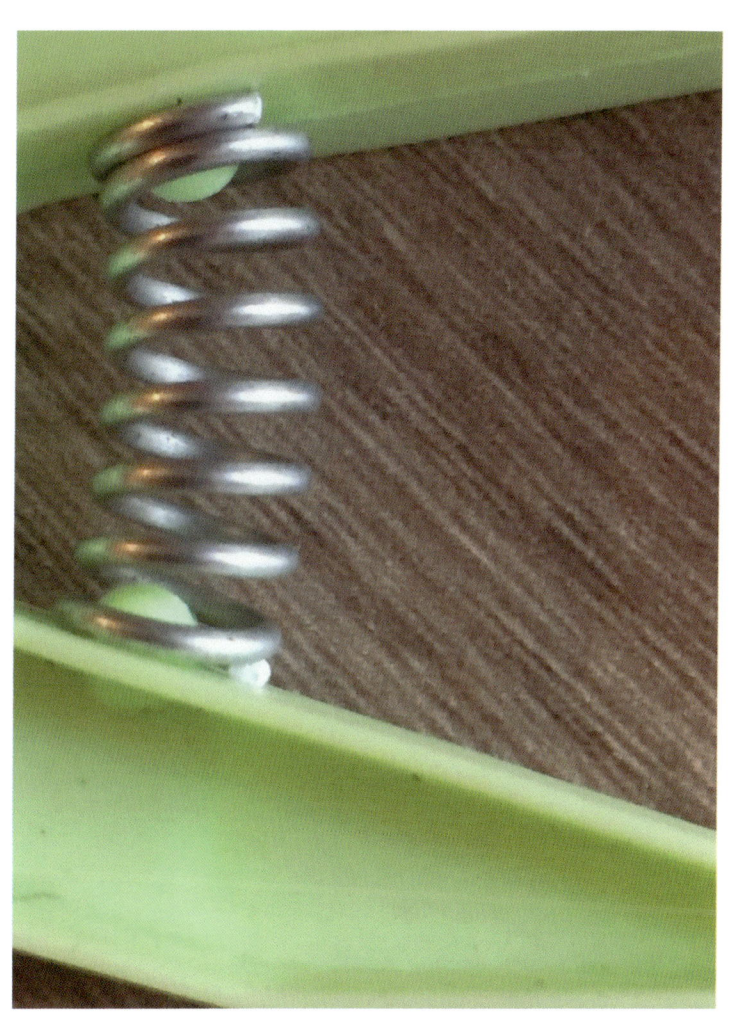

What is this?

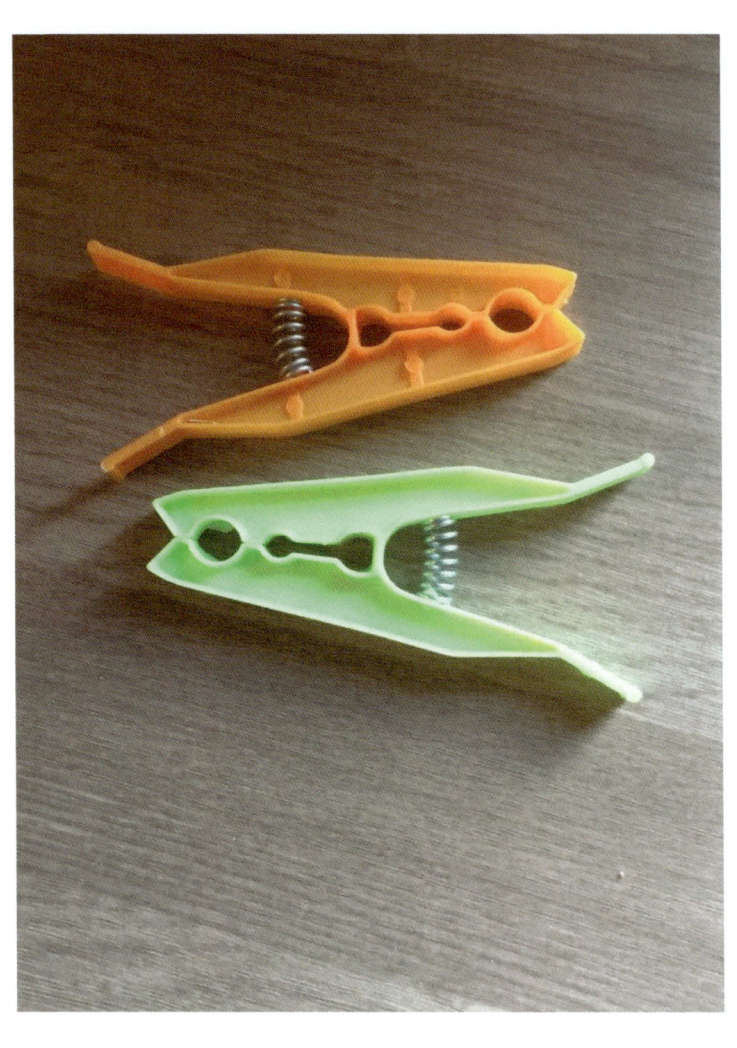

Clothes Peg

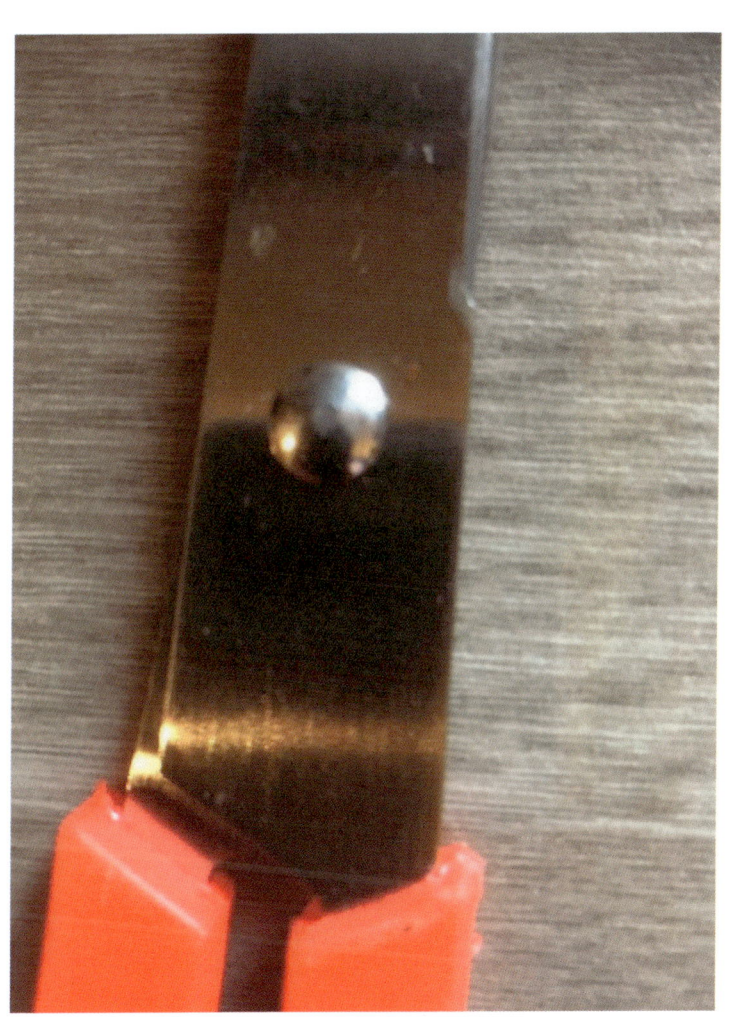

What are these?

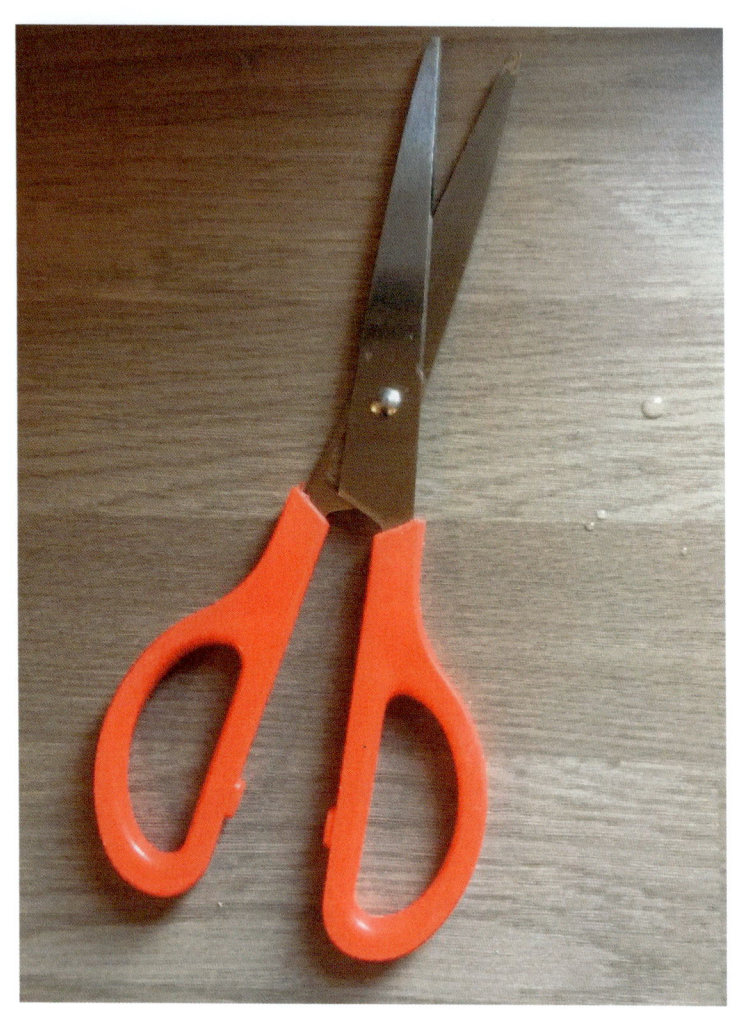

Scissors

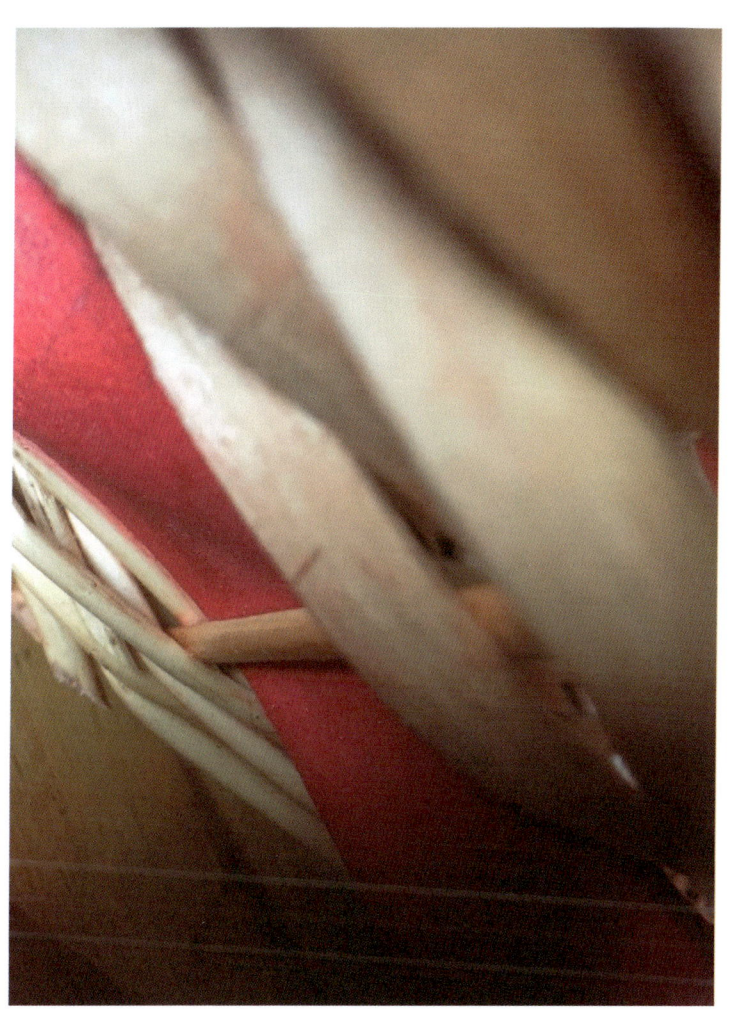

What might this be?

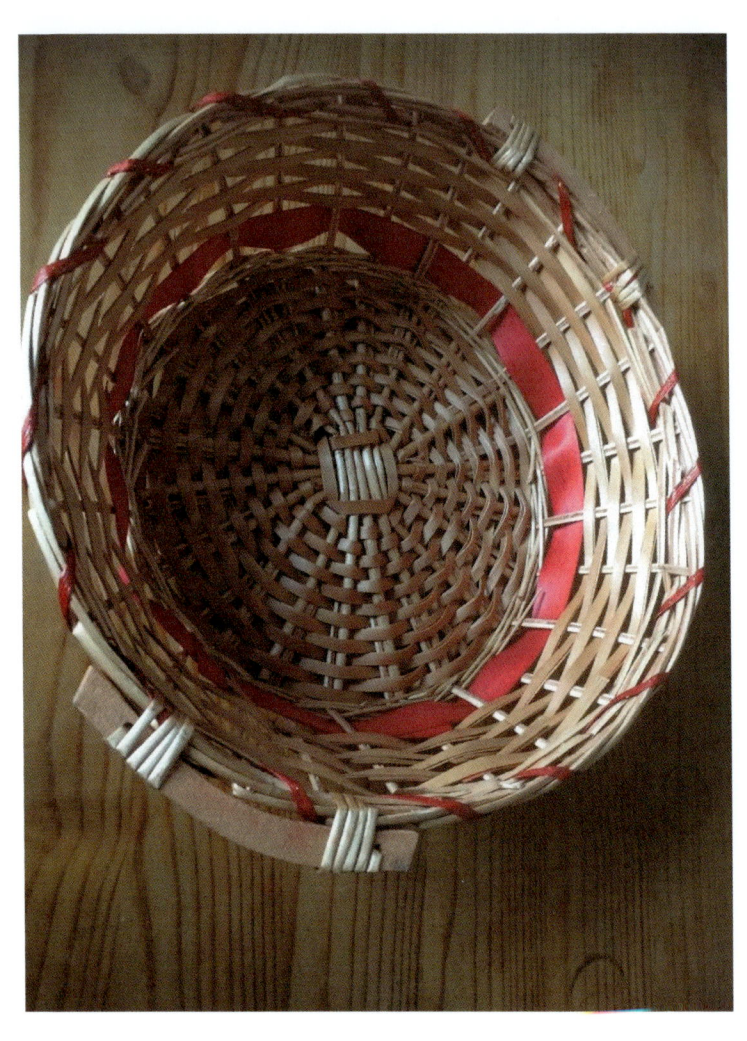

Basket

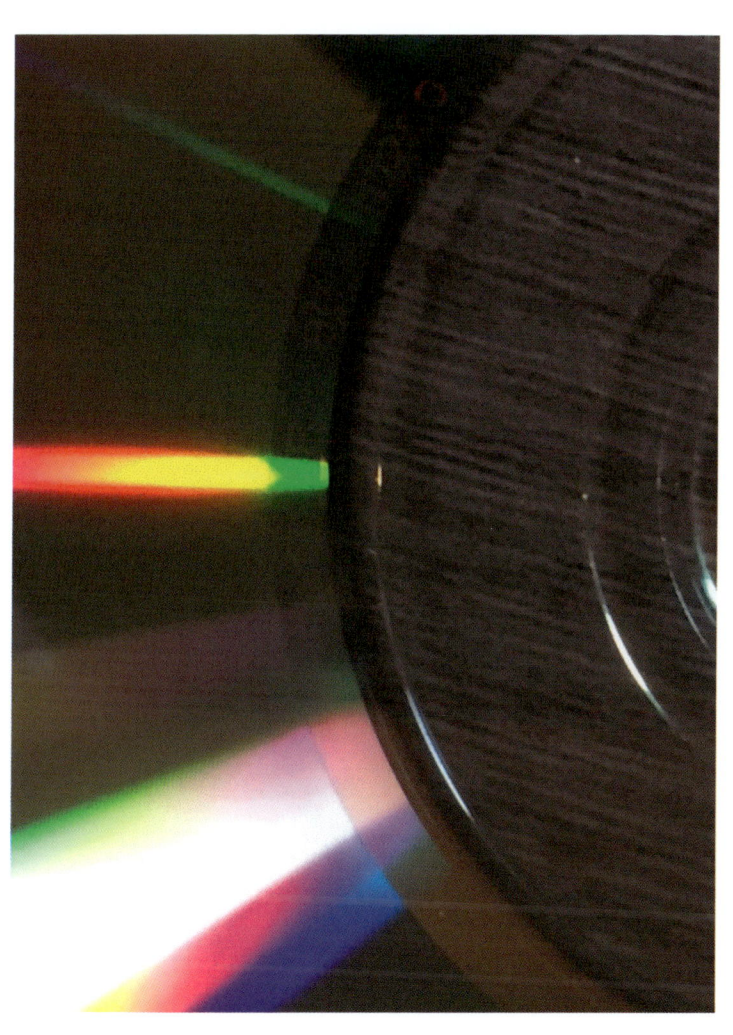

What's this?

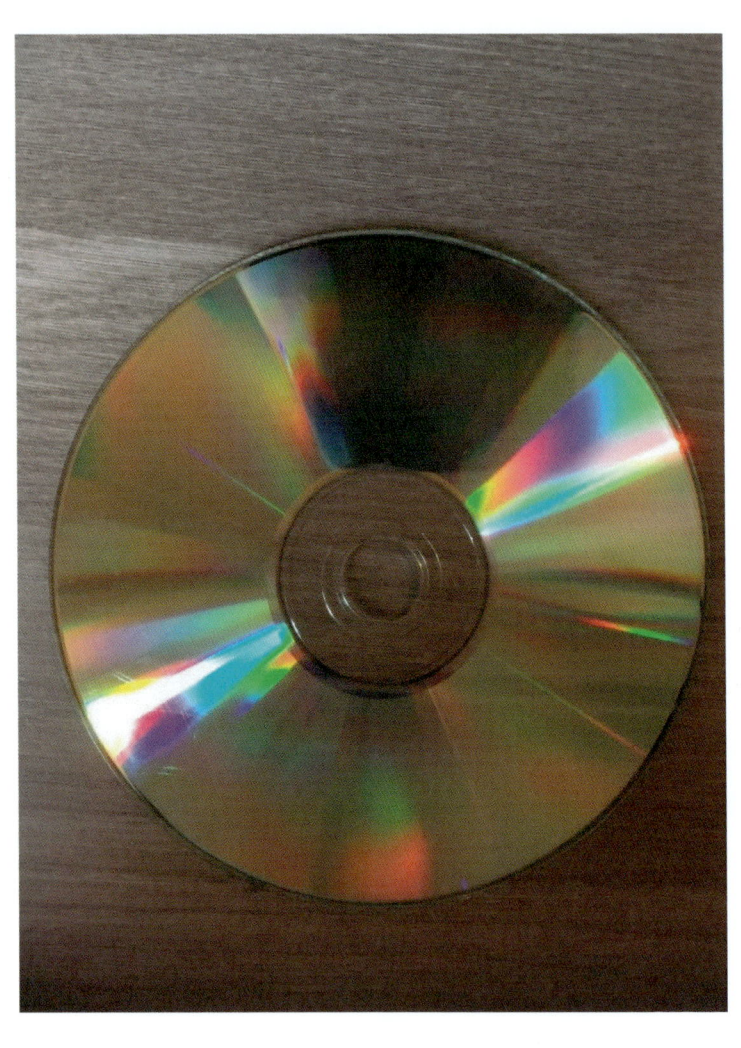

Compact Disc (CD)

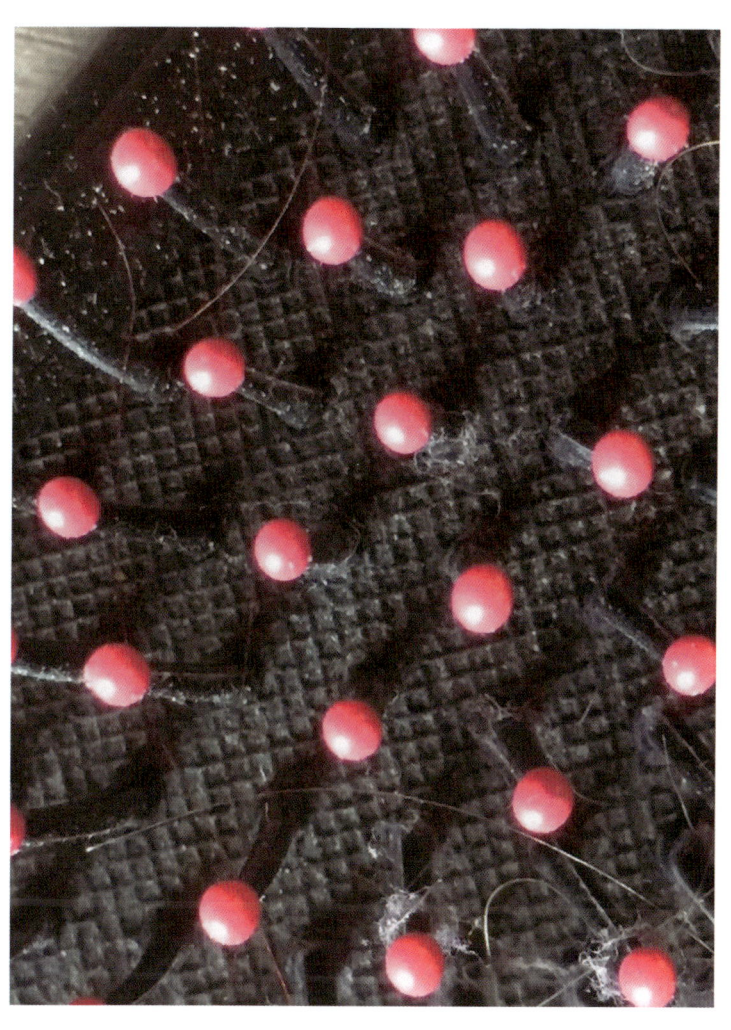

What might this be?

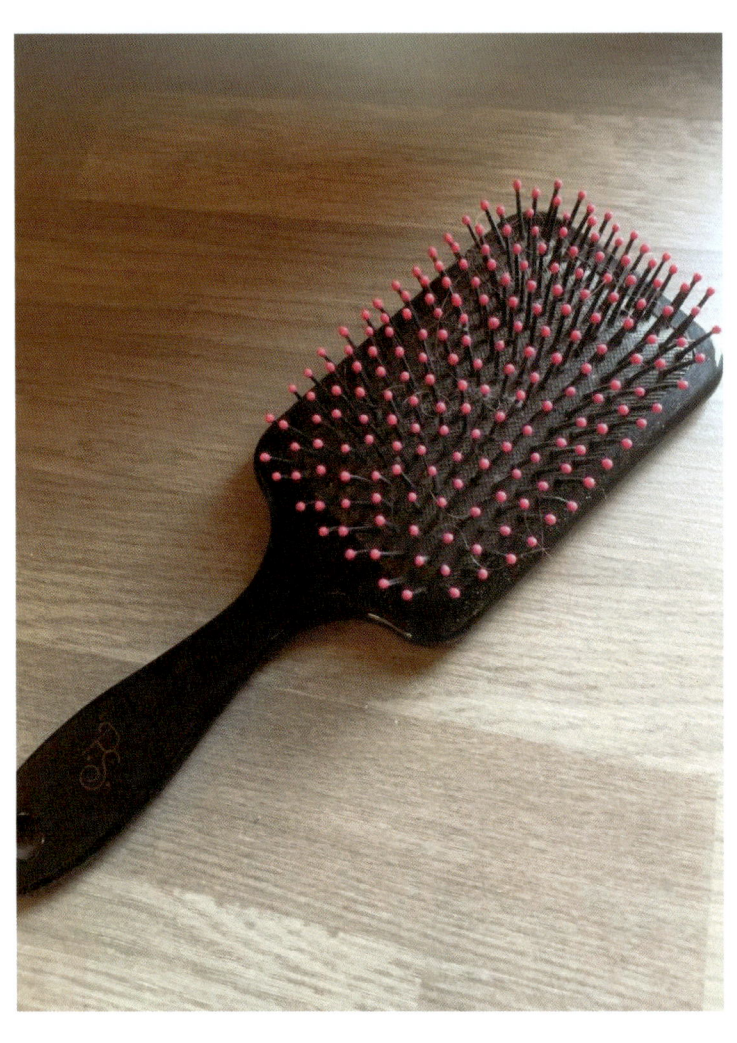

Hair Brush

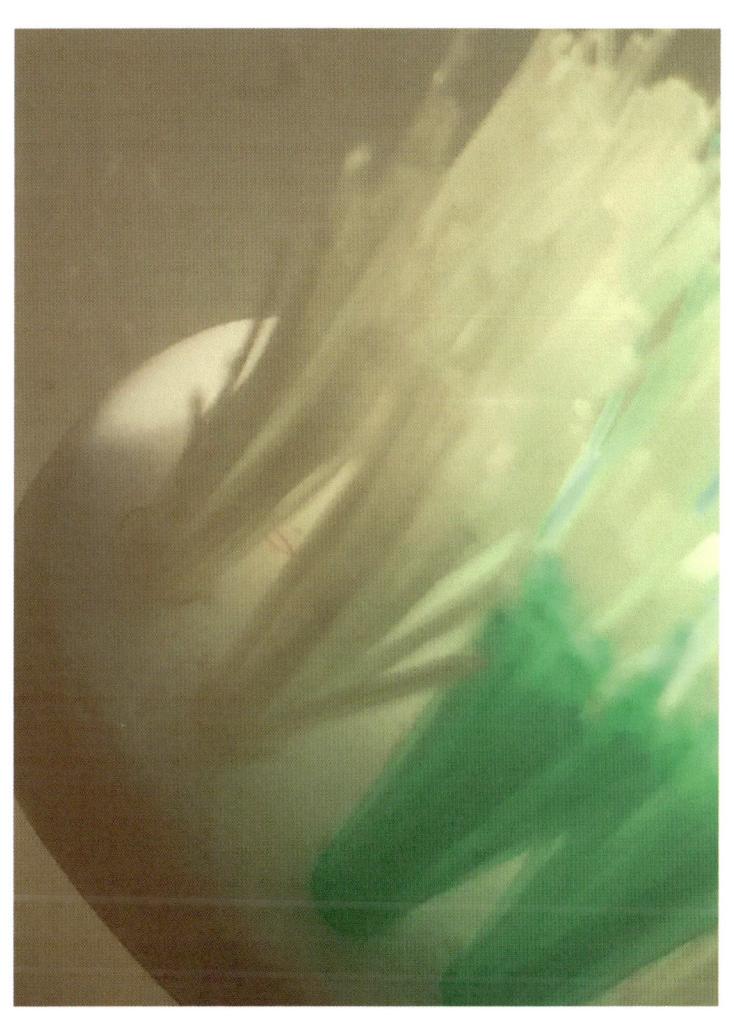

What's this?

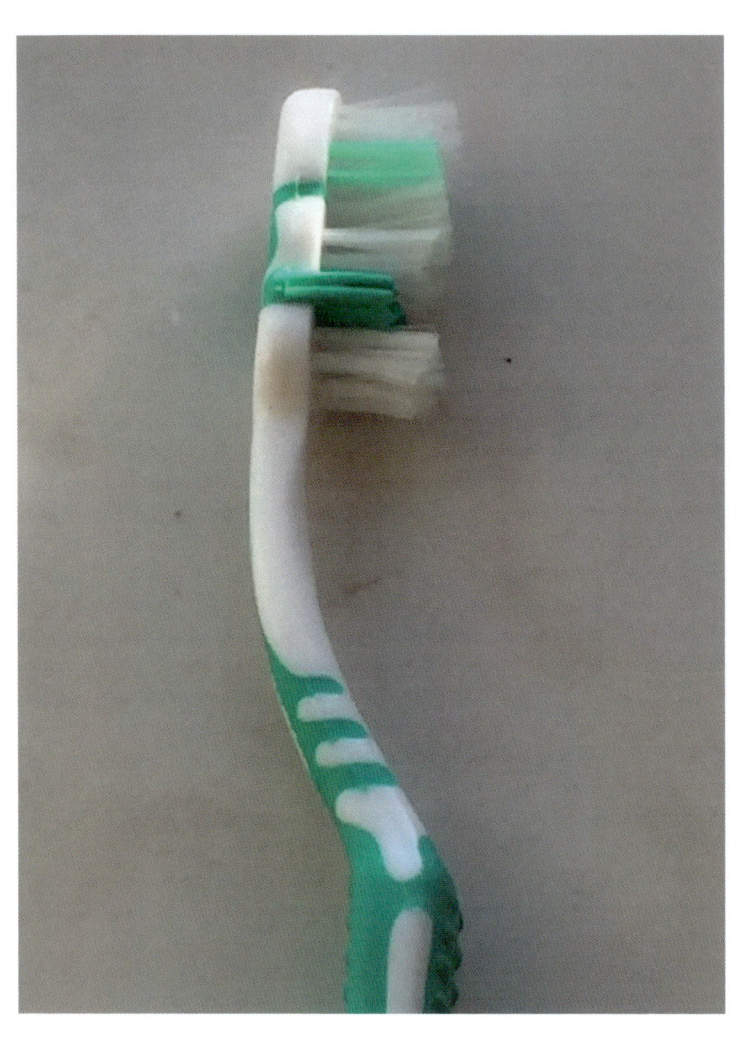

Tooth Brush

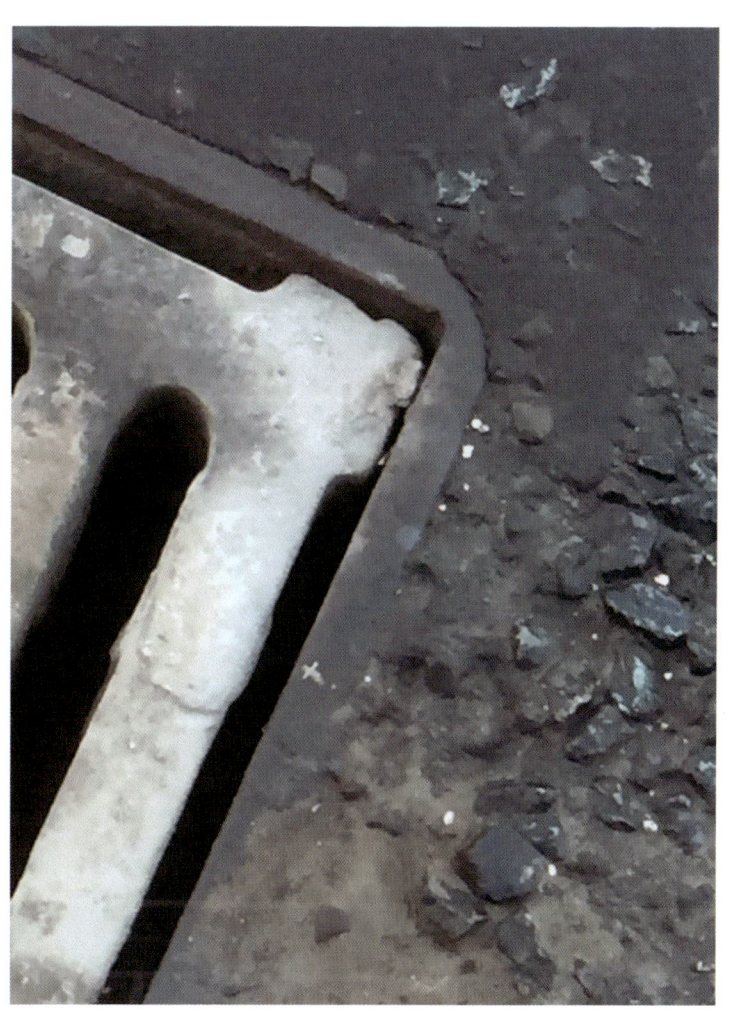

What is this?

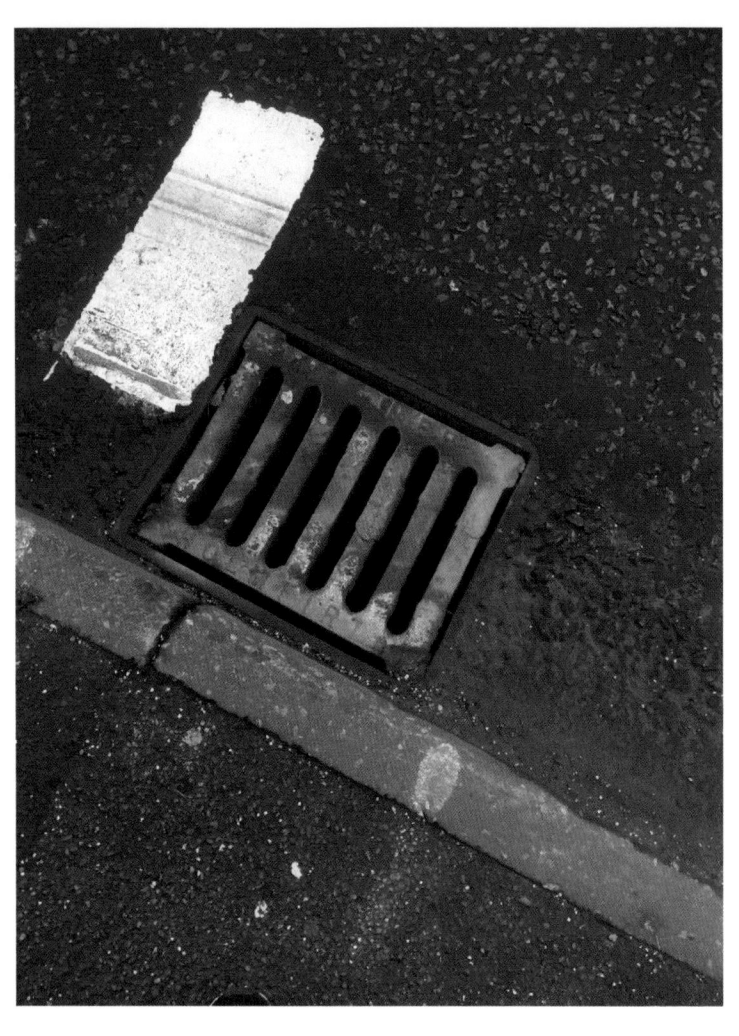

Drain

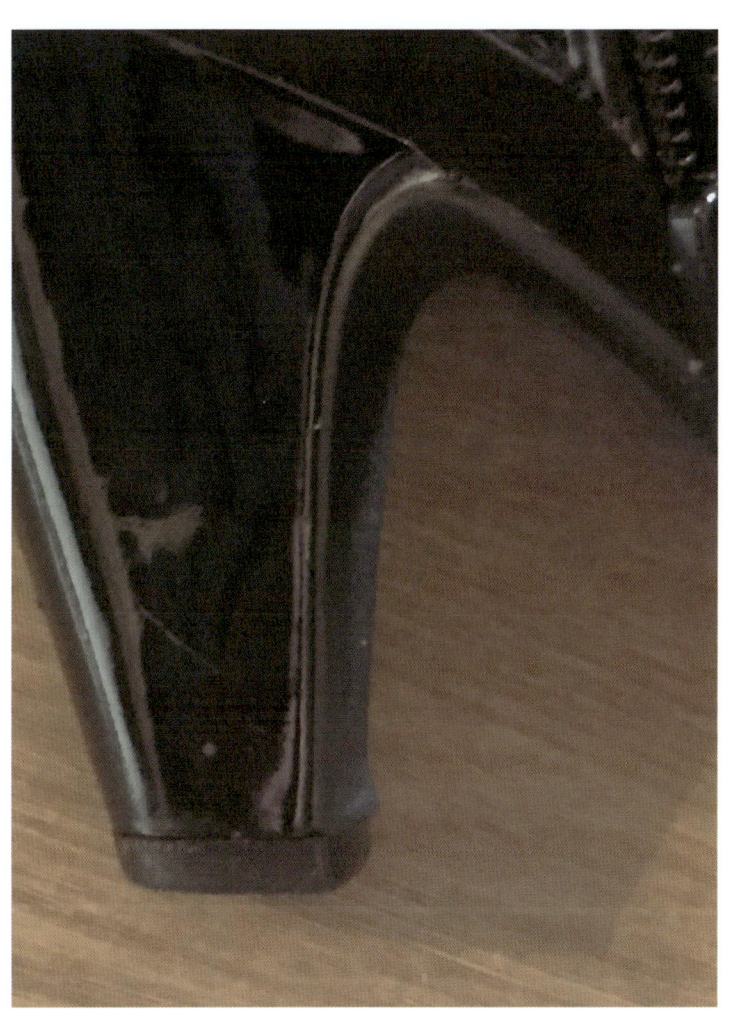

What might this be?

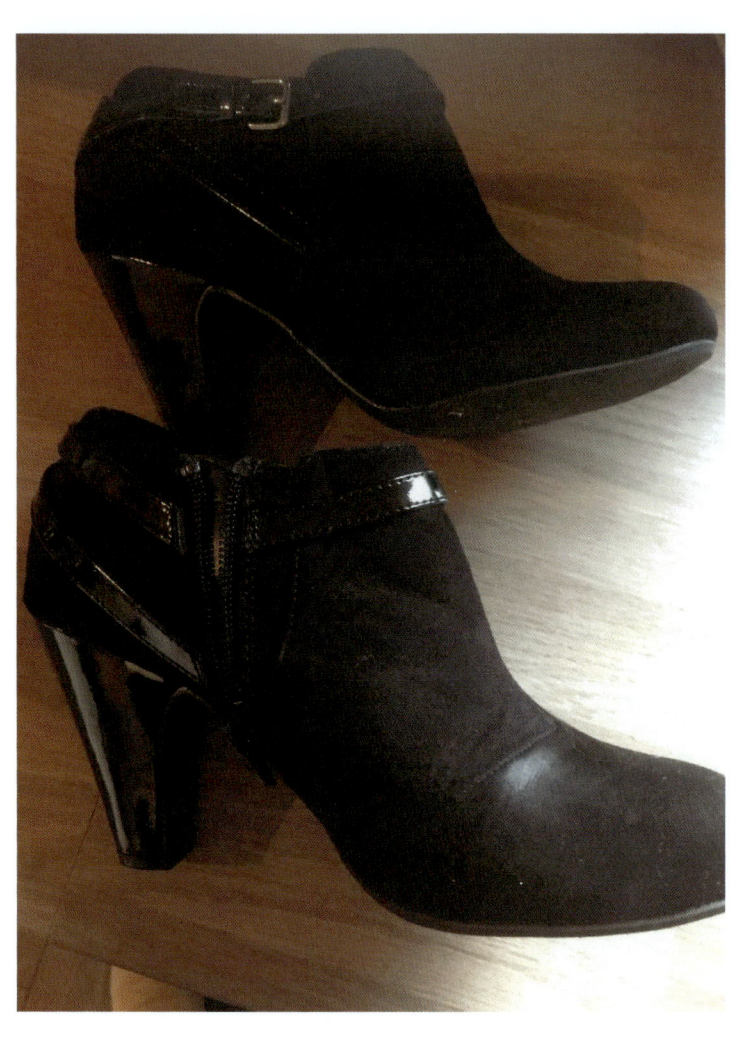

Ladies Boots

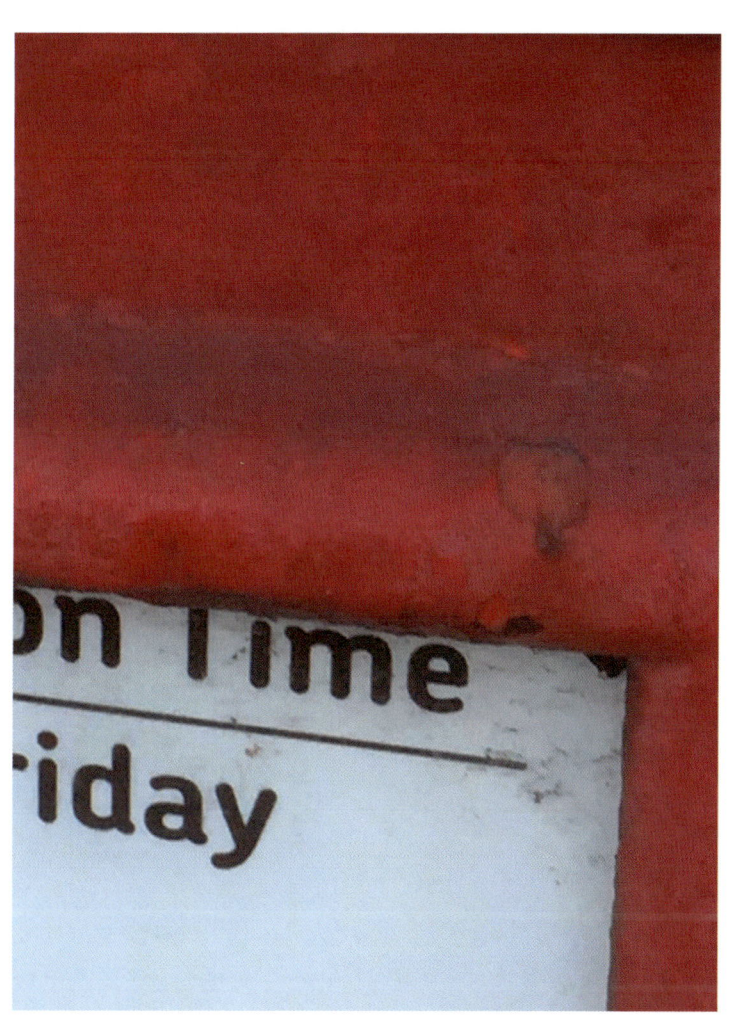

What could this be?

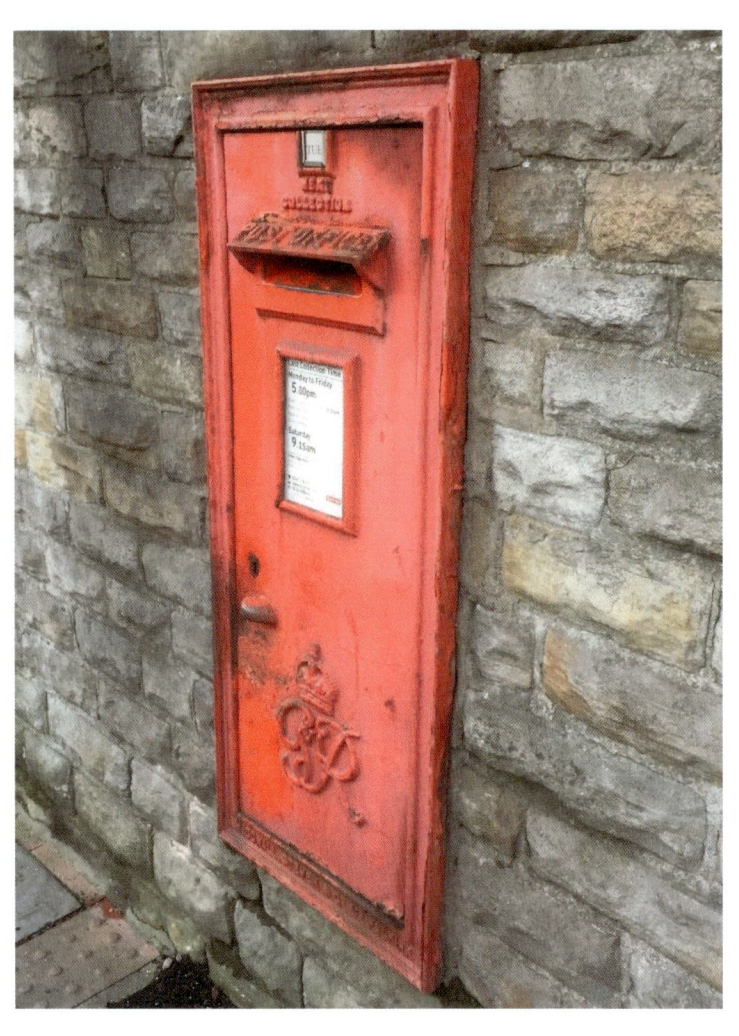

Post Box

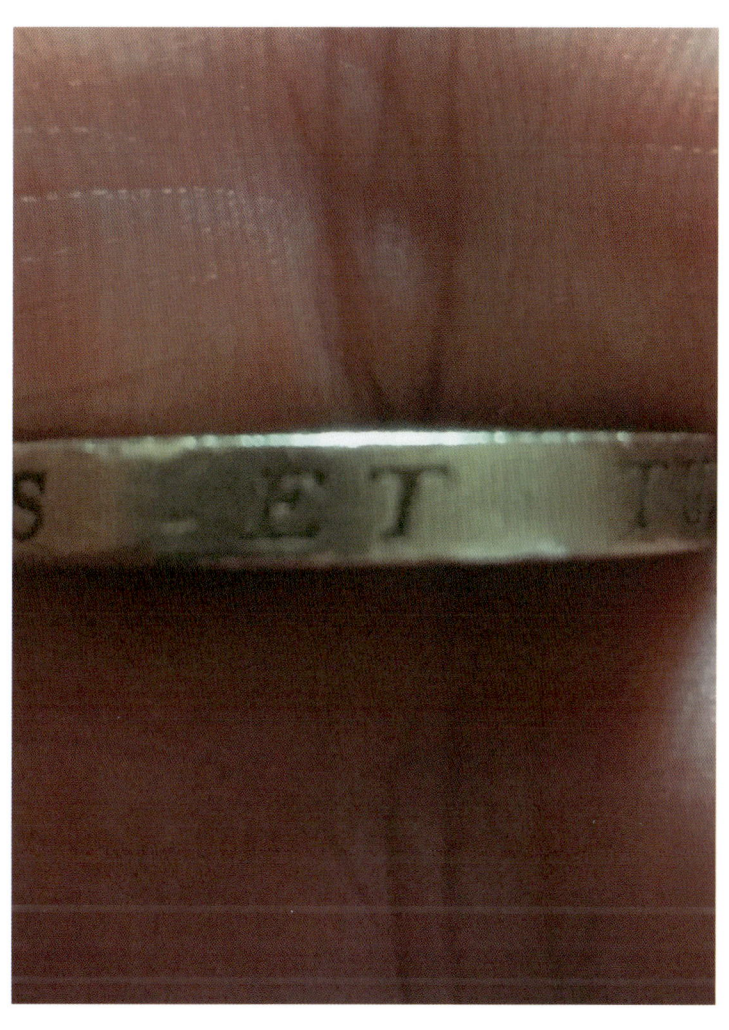

Do you recognise this?

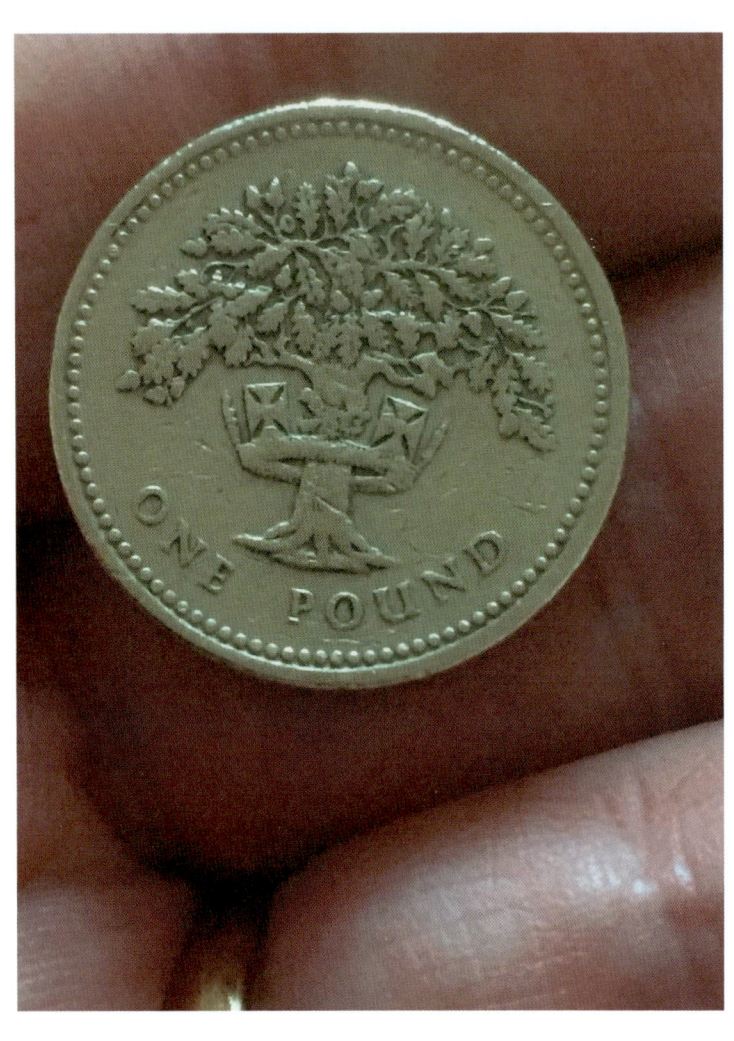

One Pound Coin

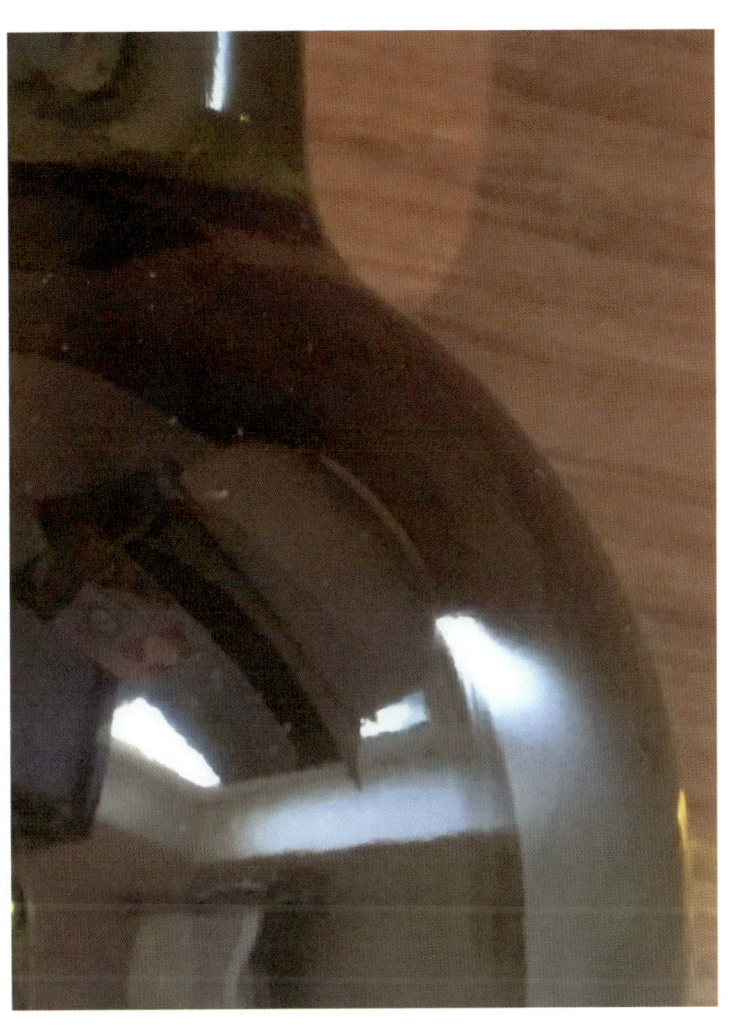

What is this?

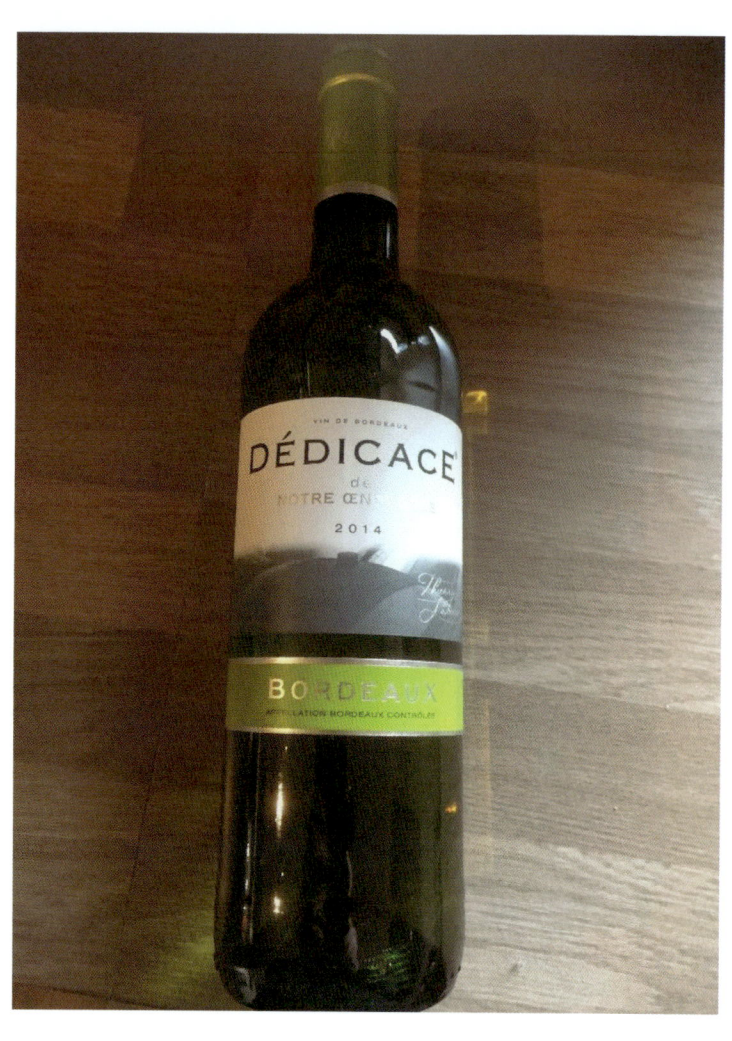

A bottle of wine

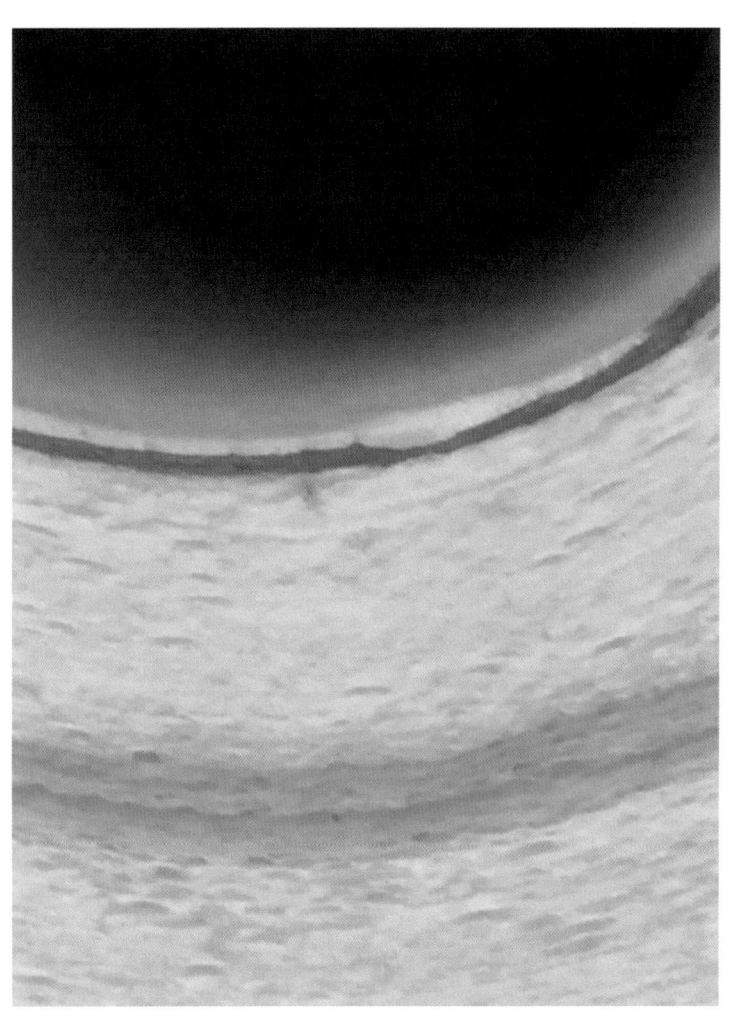

What's this?

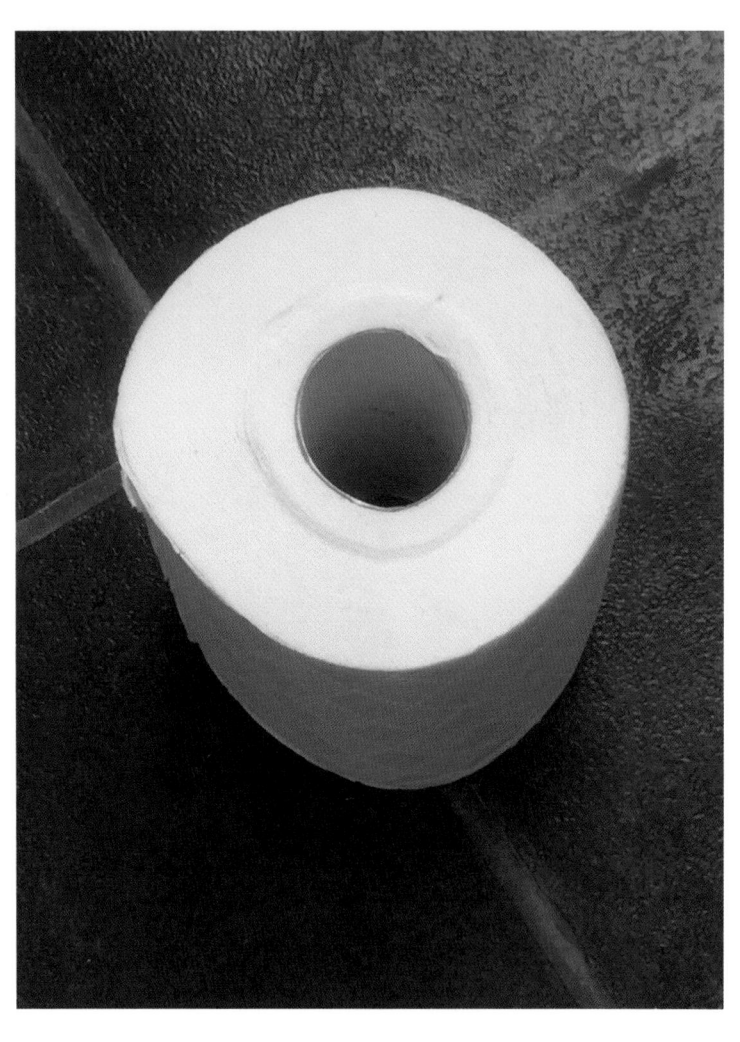

Toilet Roll

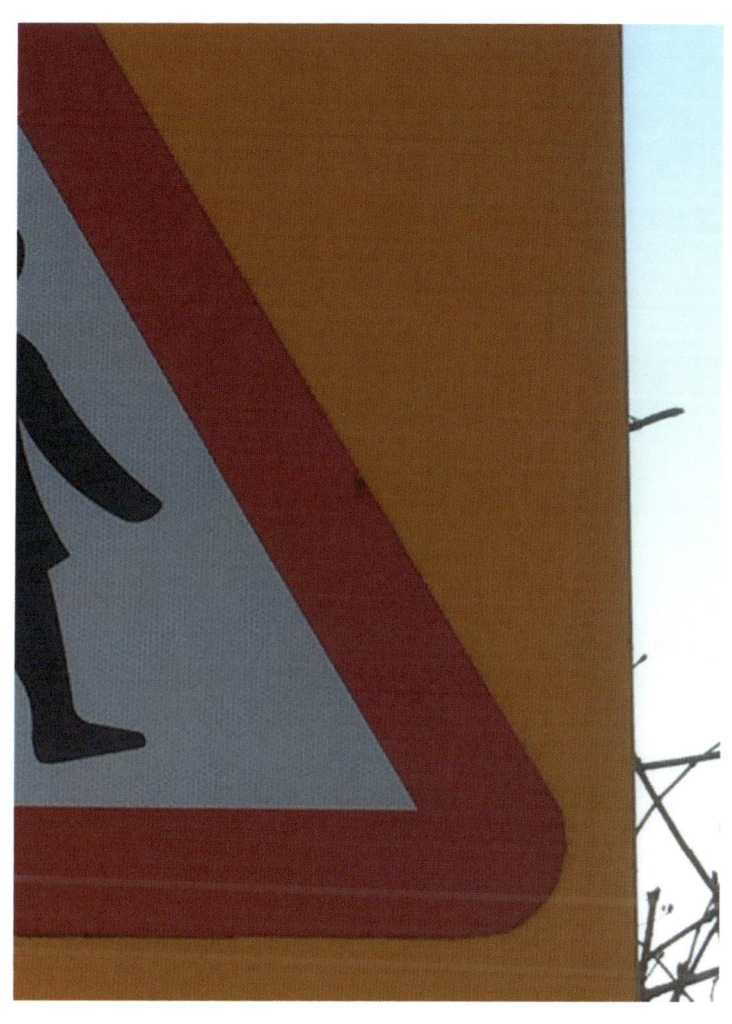

Do you recognise this?

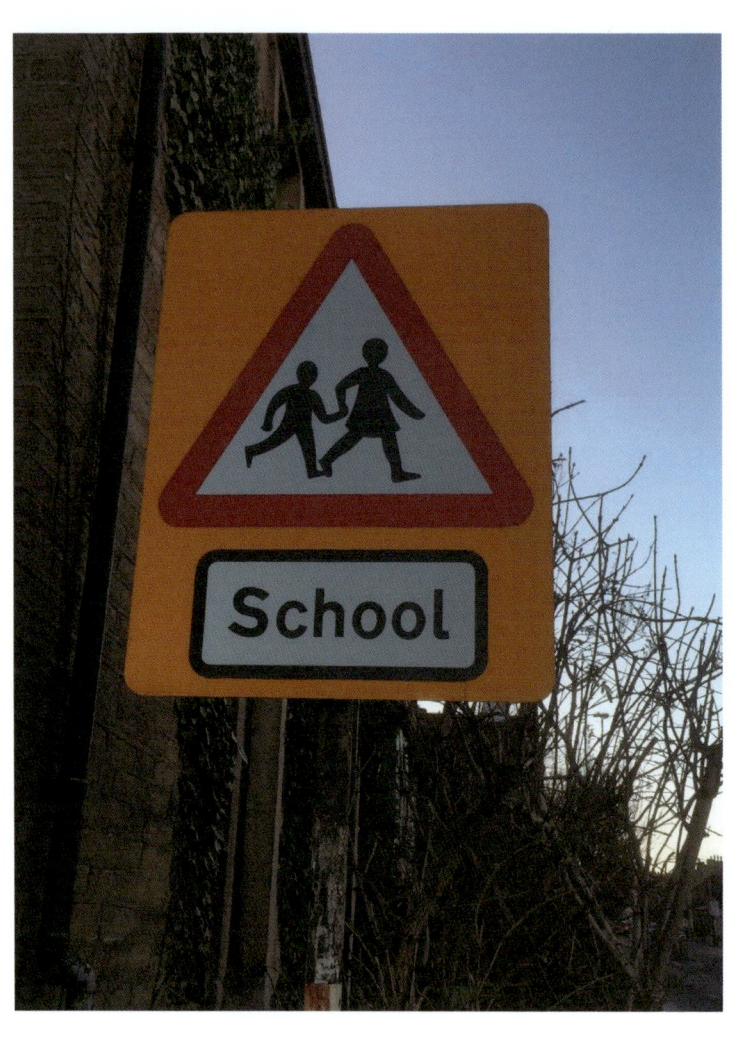

Road Sign

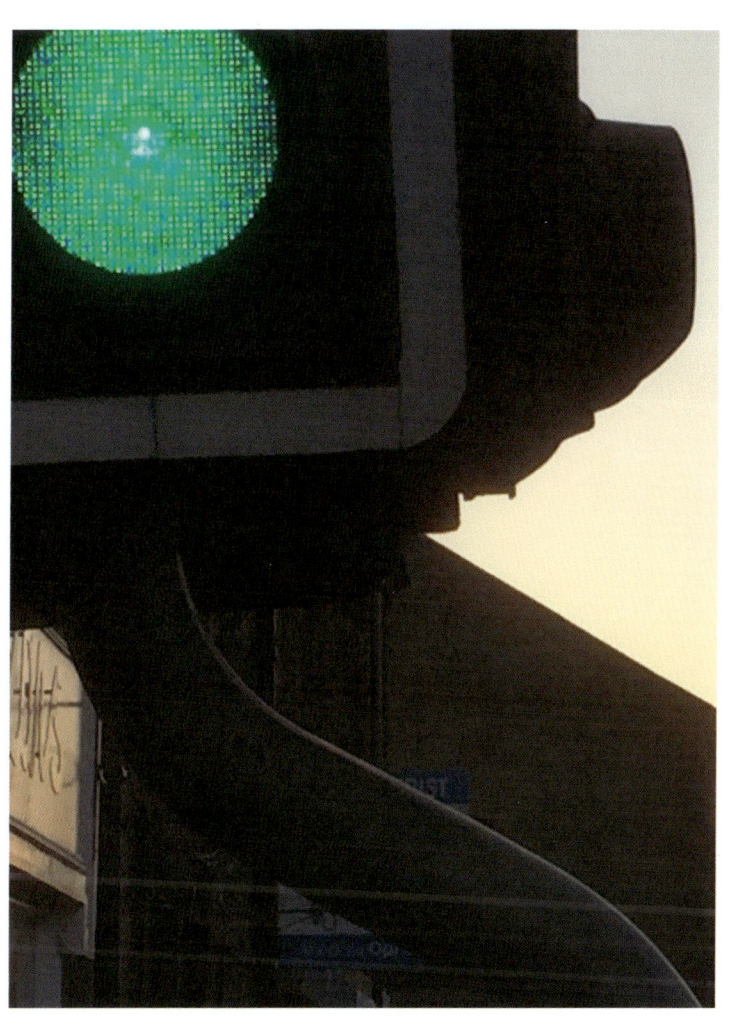

Recognise?

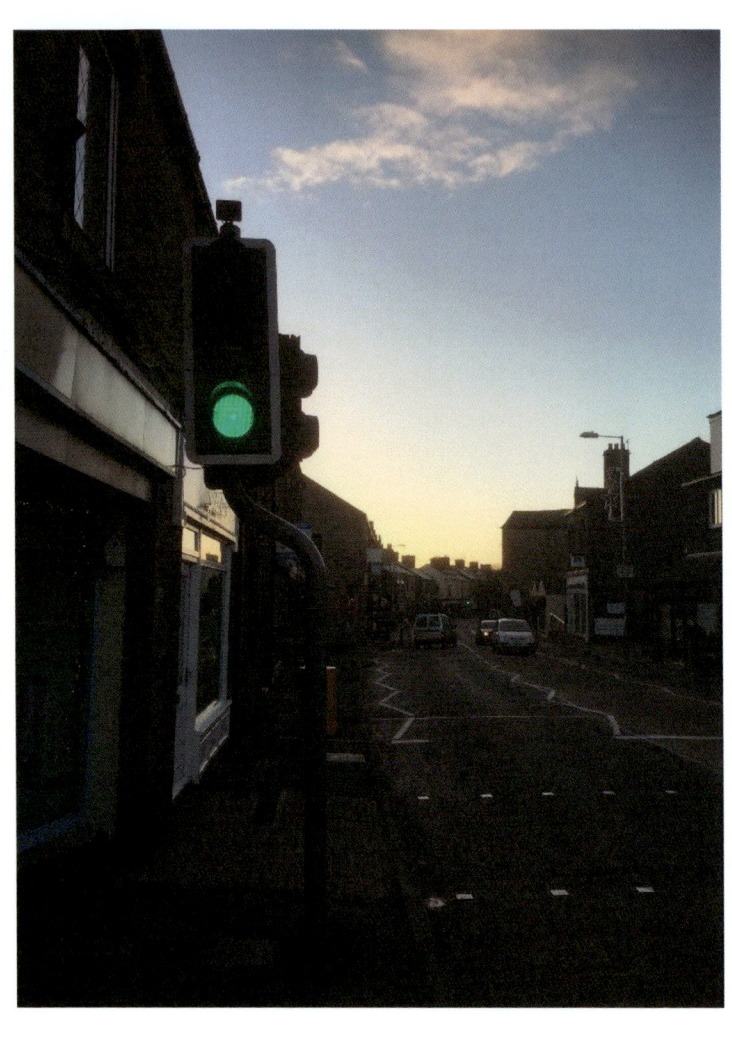

Traffic Light

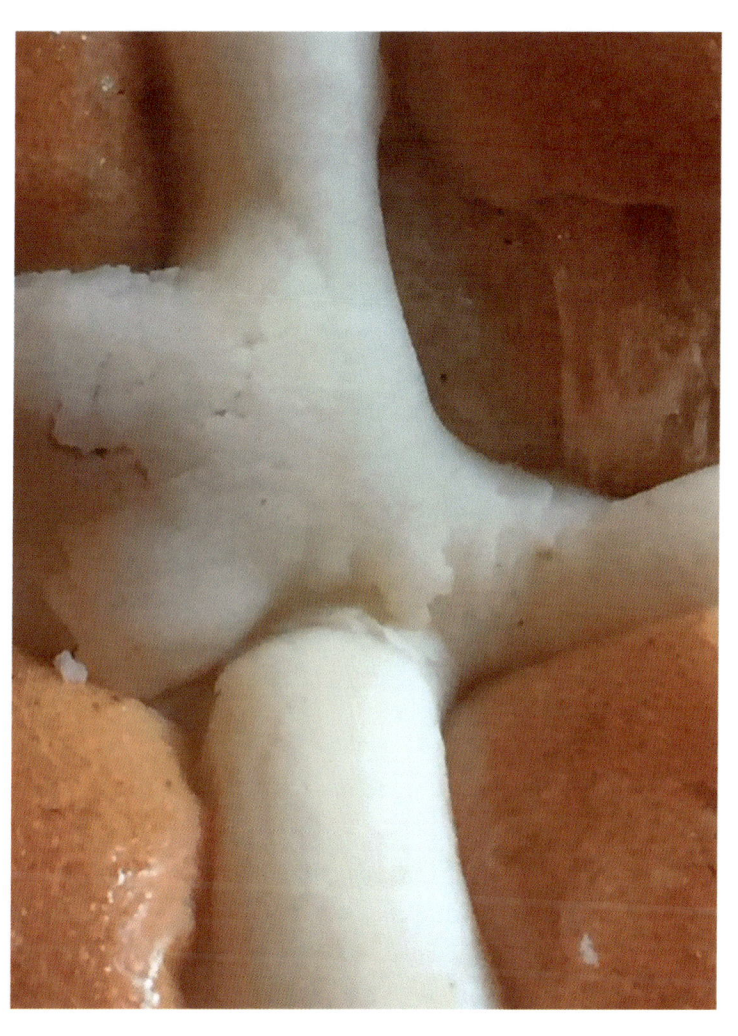

What is this?

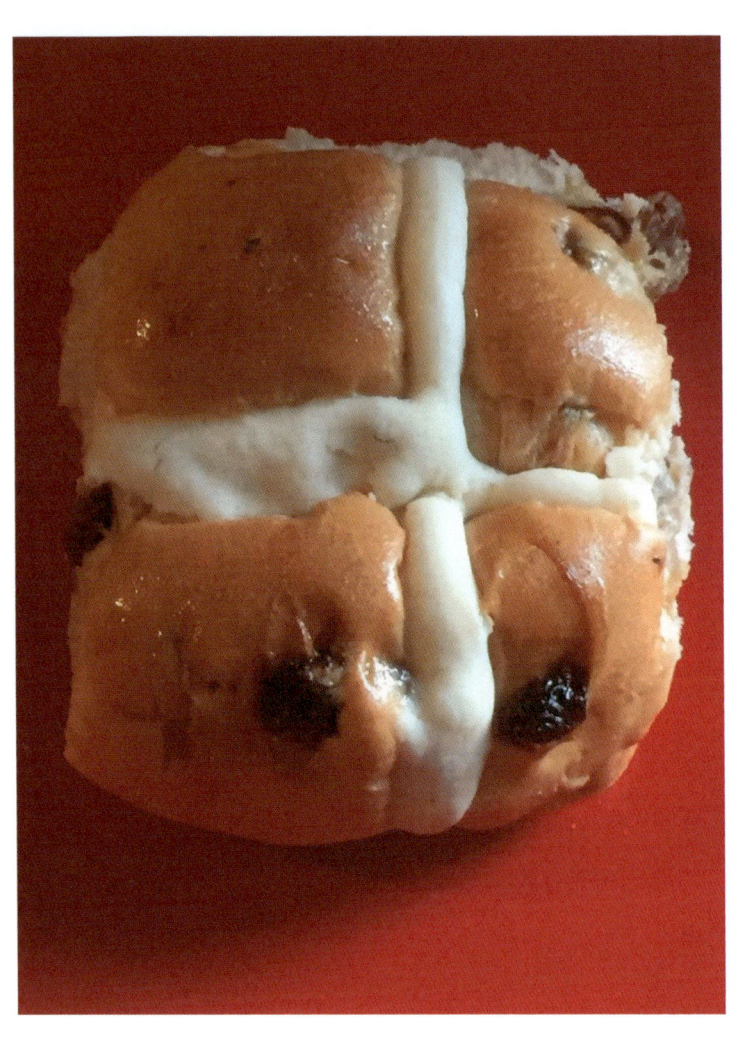

Hot Cross Bun

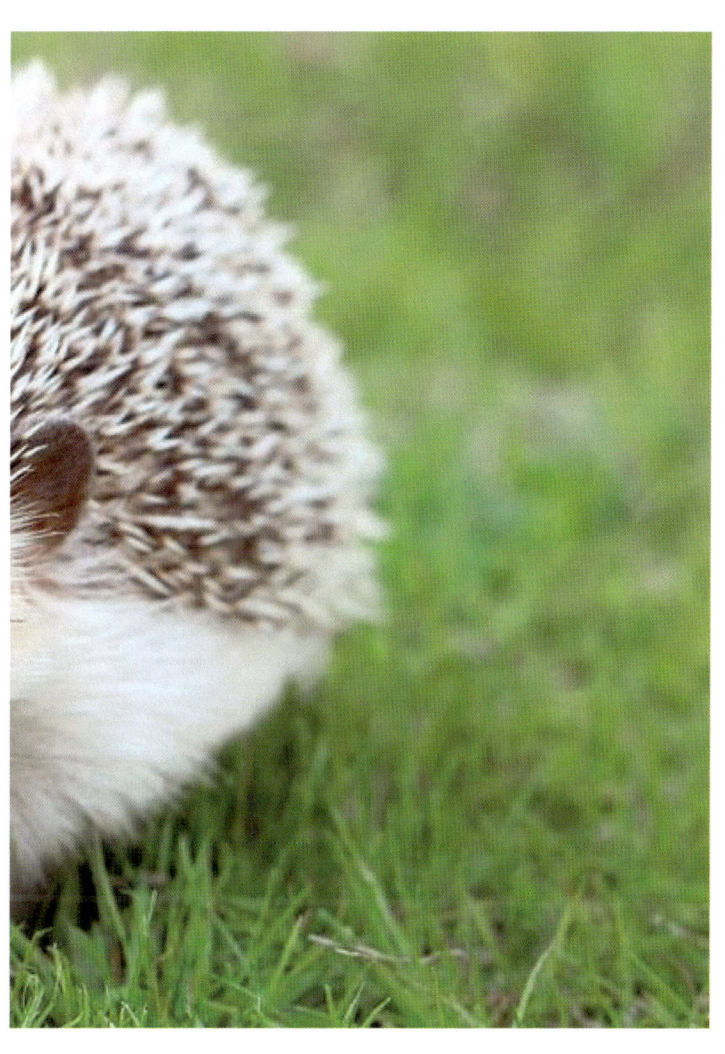

What is this?

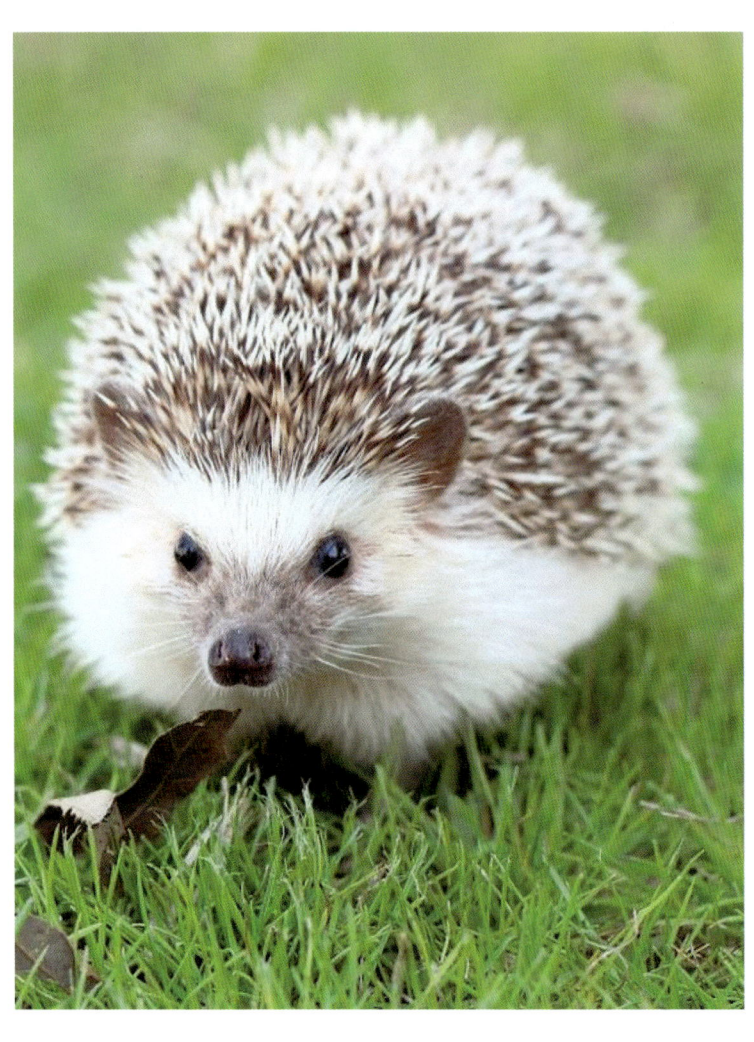

Hedgehog

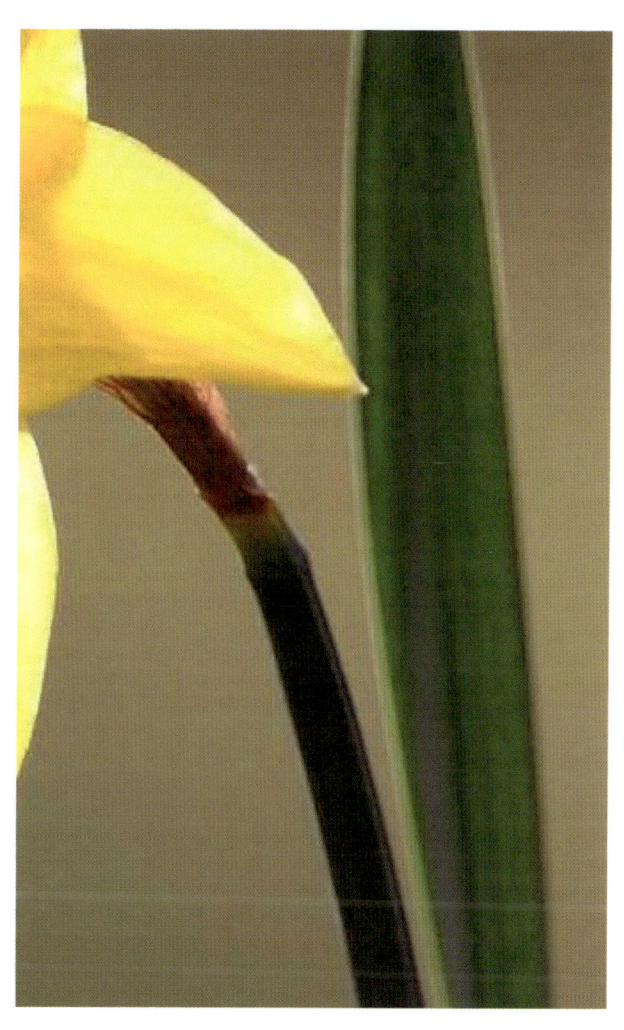

What is this?

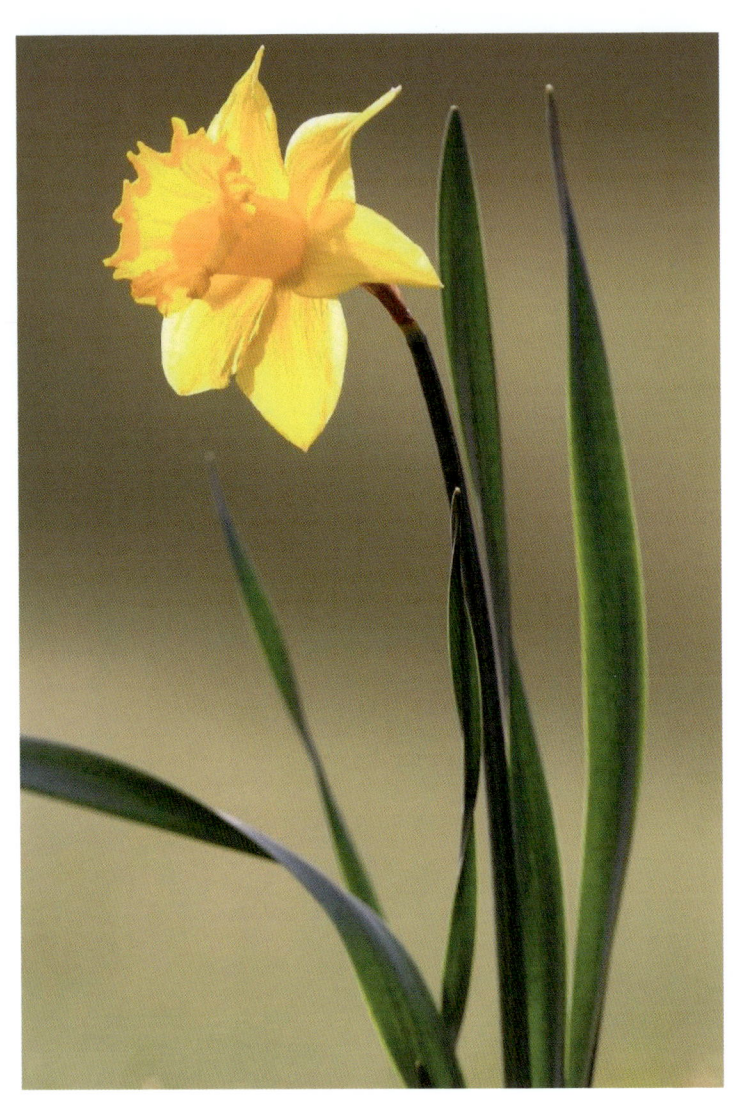

Daffodil

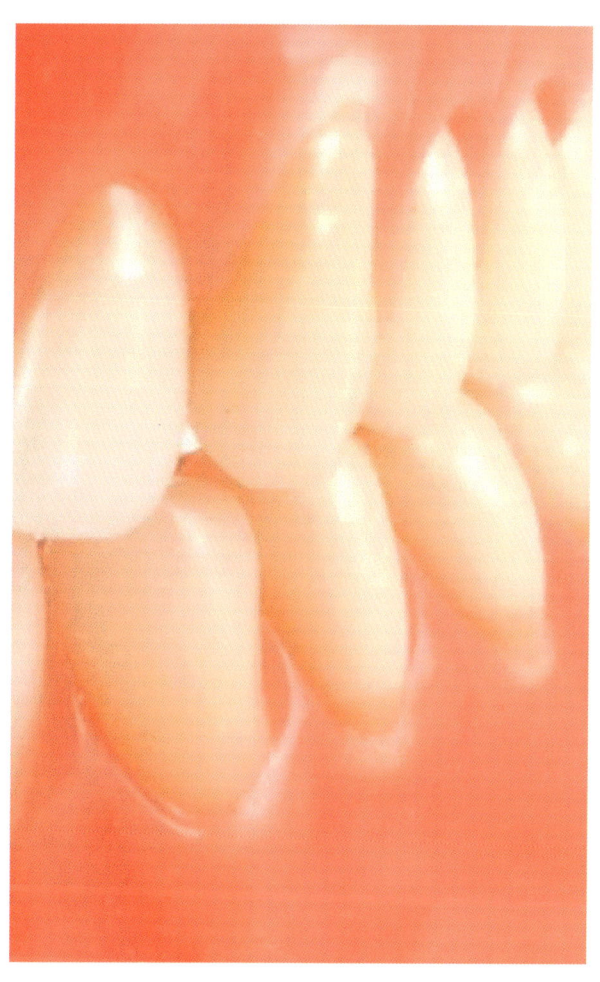

What are these?

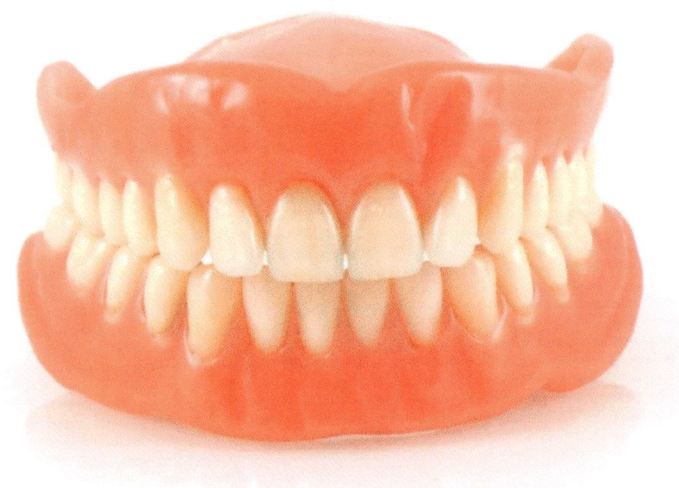

False Teeth

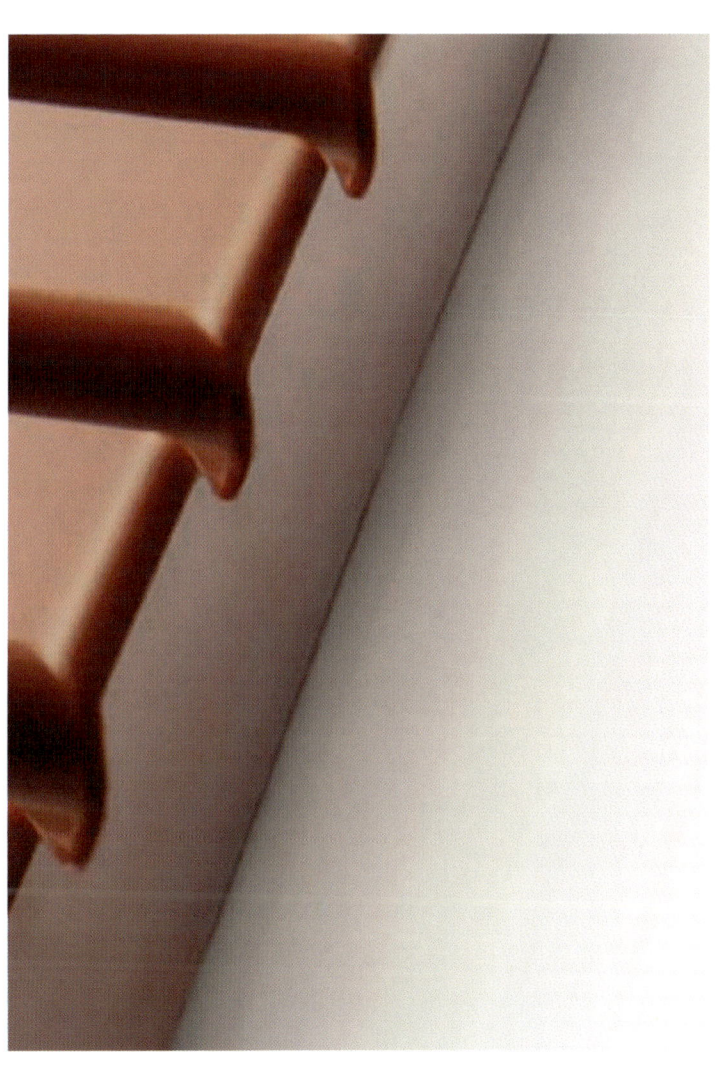

What is this?

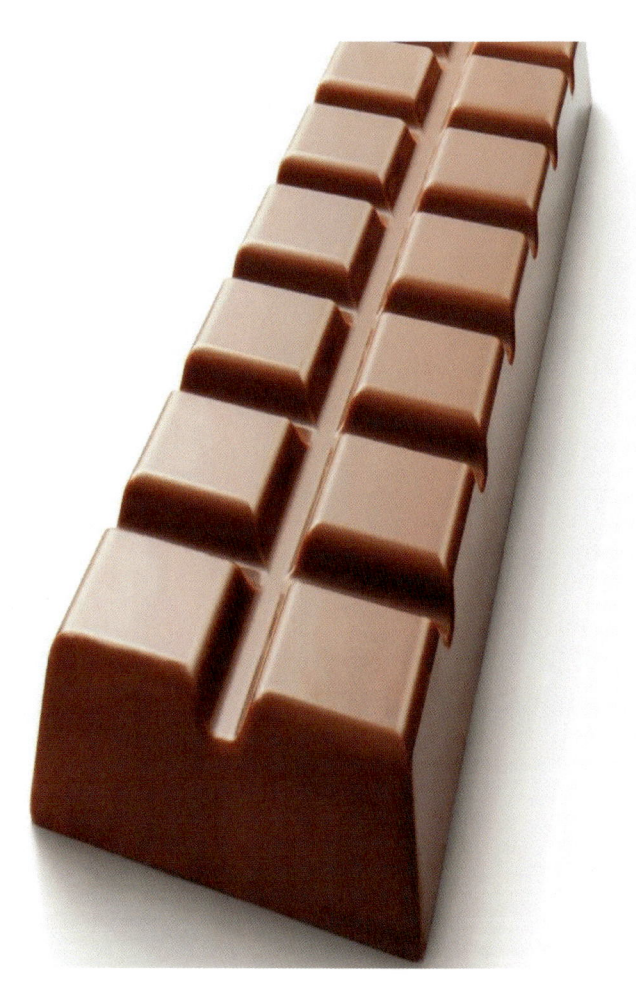

Chocolate Bar

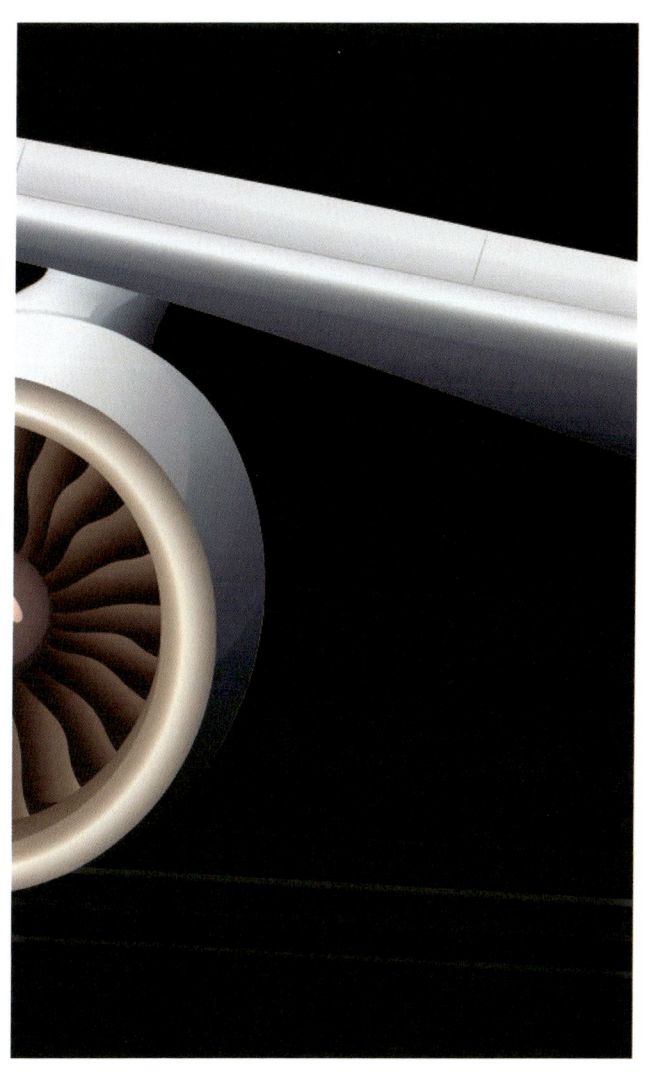

What is this part of?

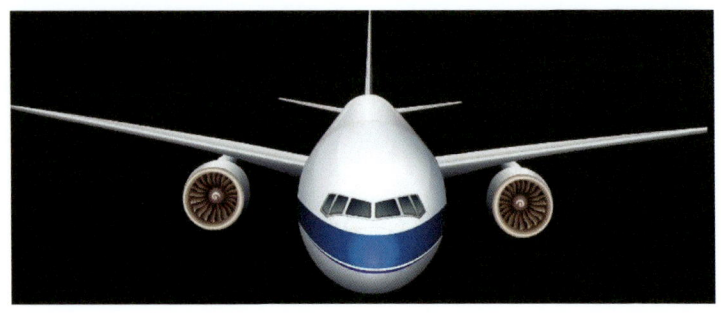

Aeroplane

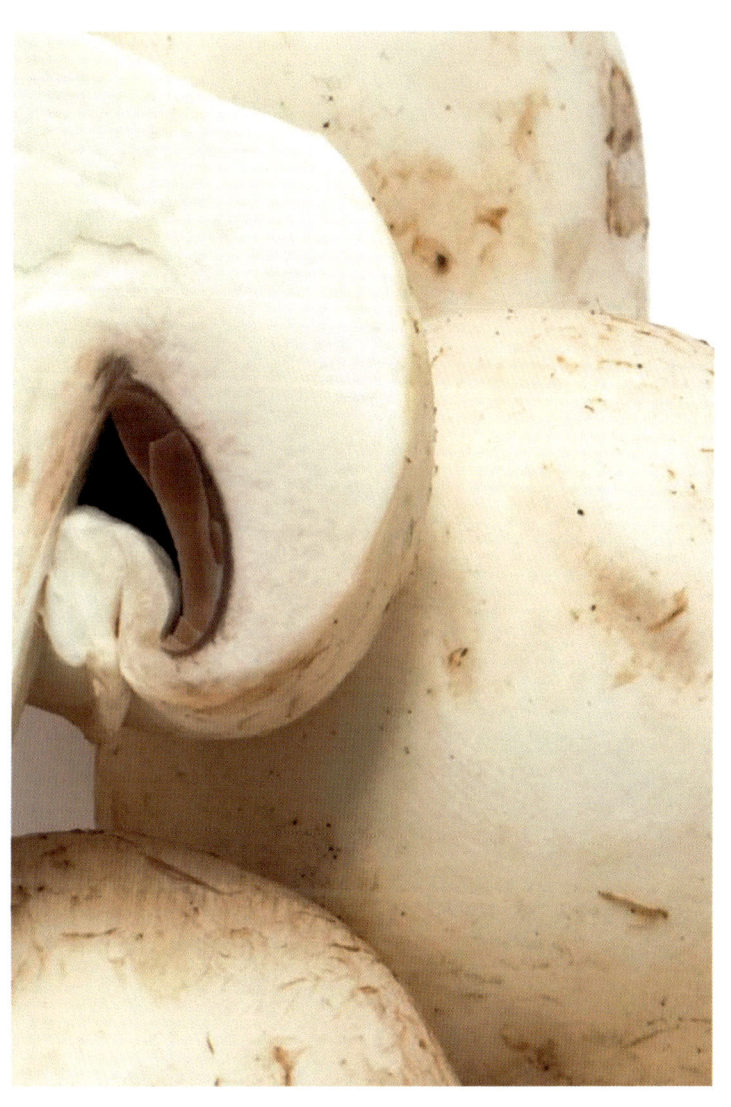

What are these?

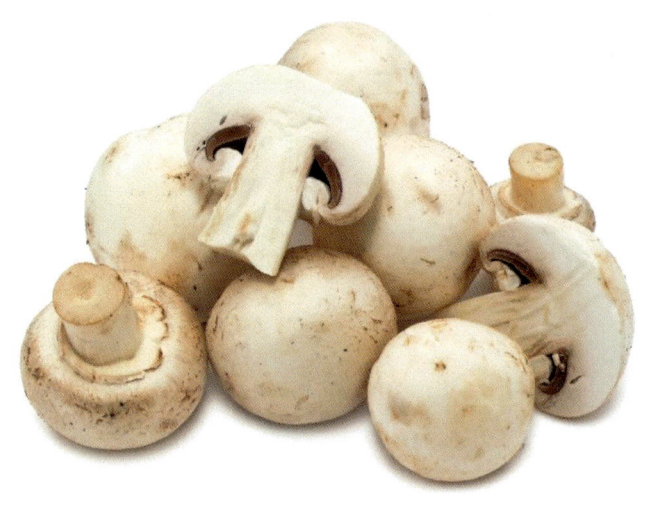

Mushrooms

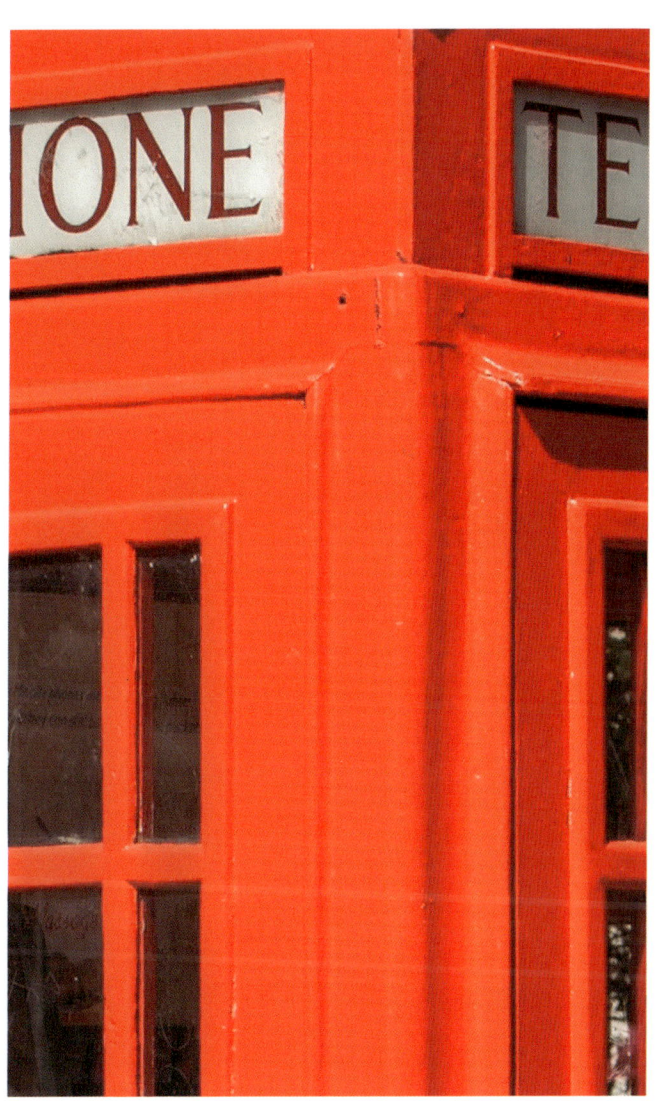

What is this?

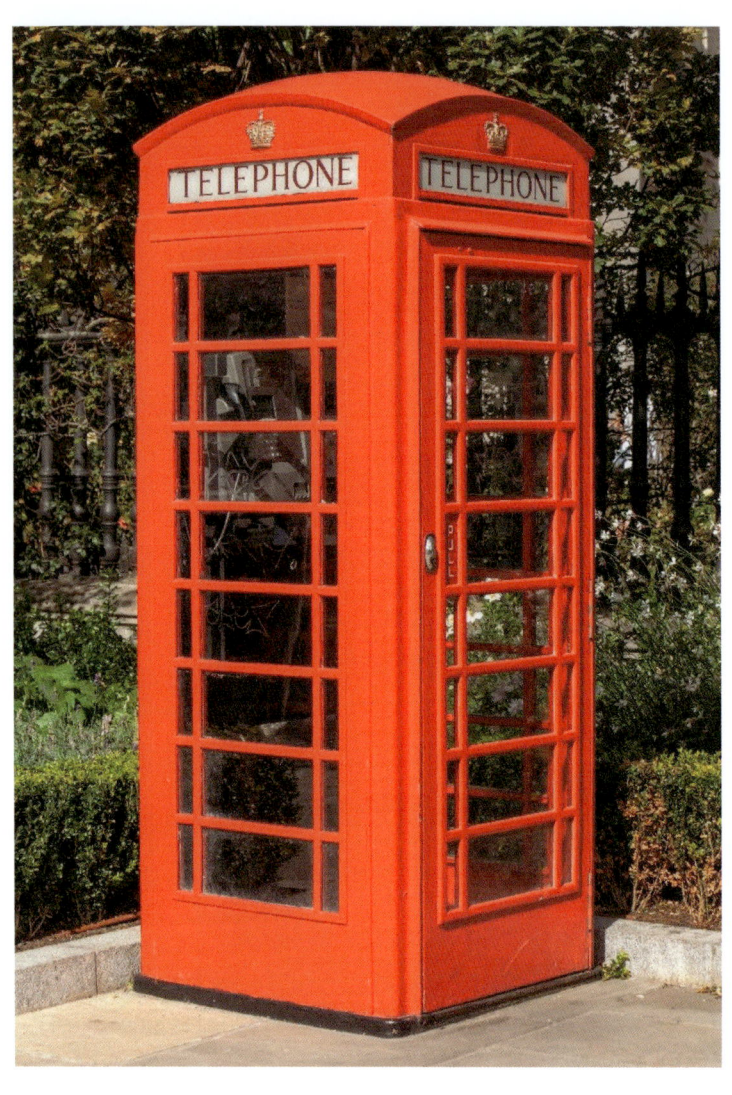

Telephone Box

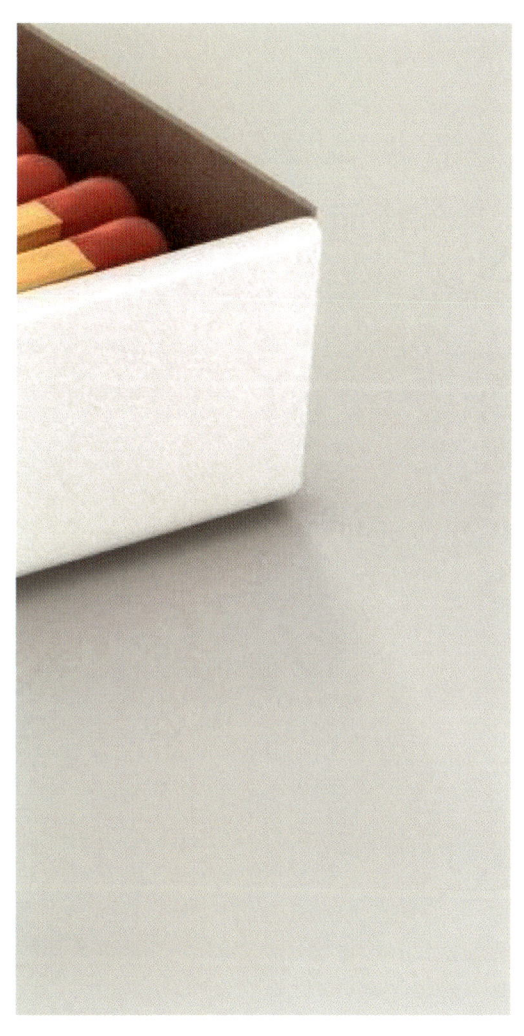

What are these?

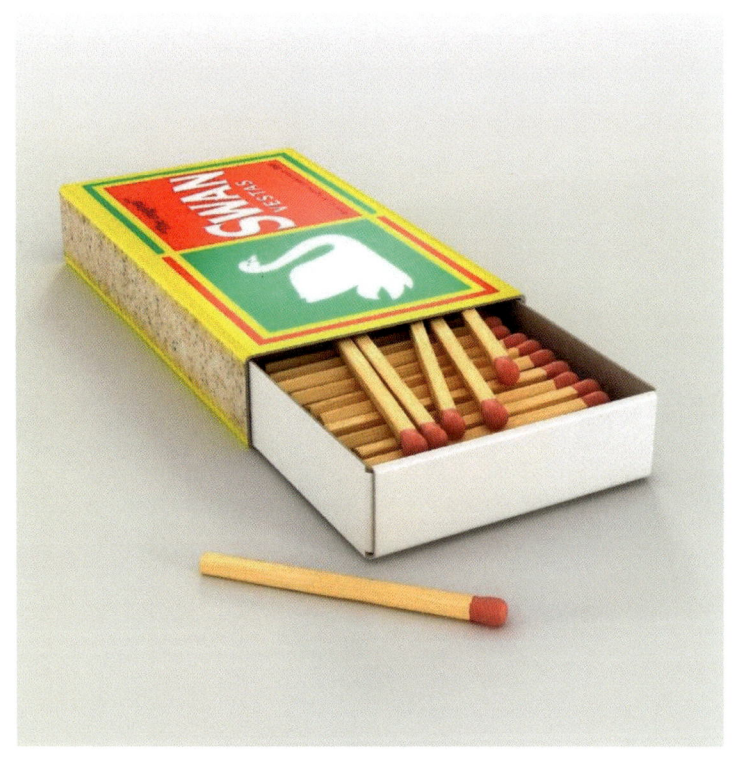

Matches

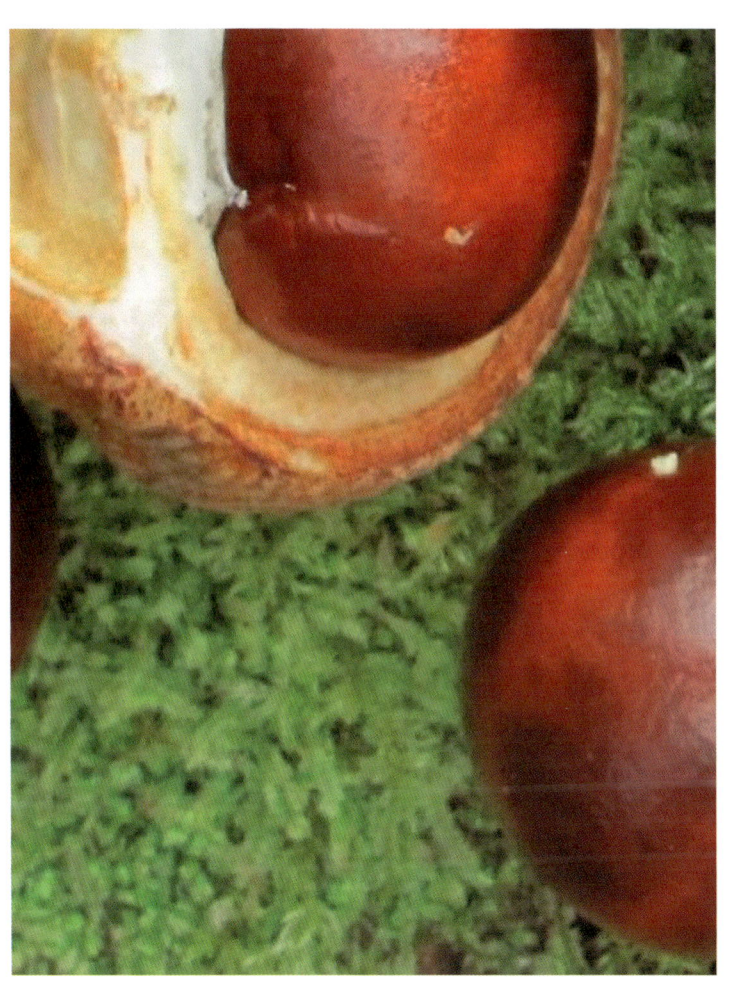

What are these?

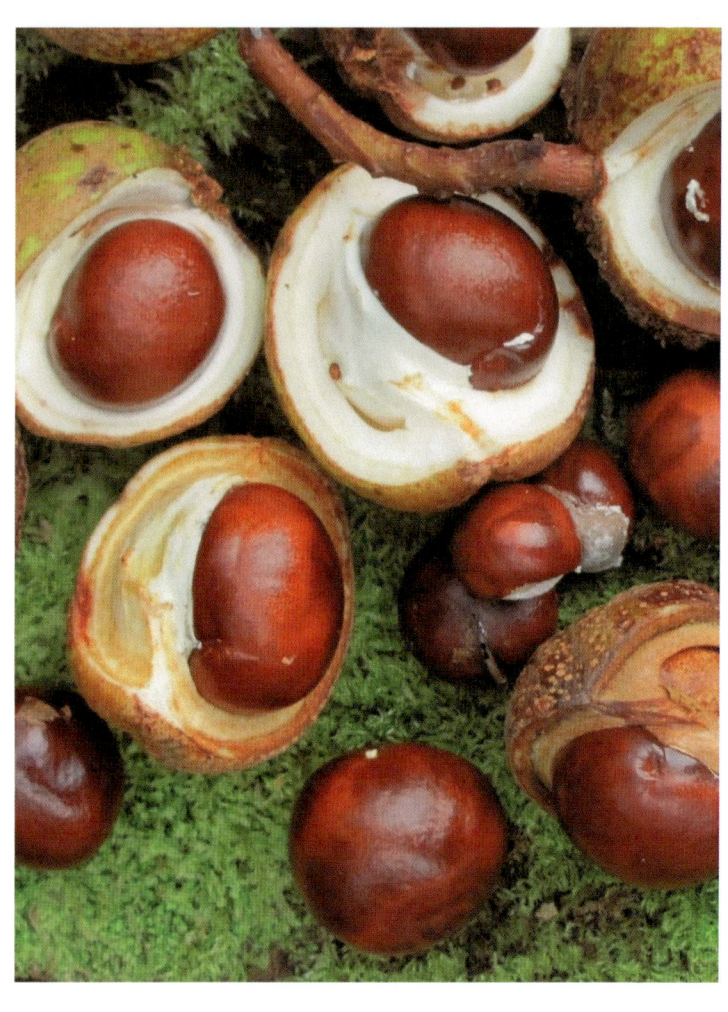

Conkers

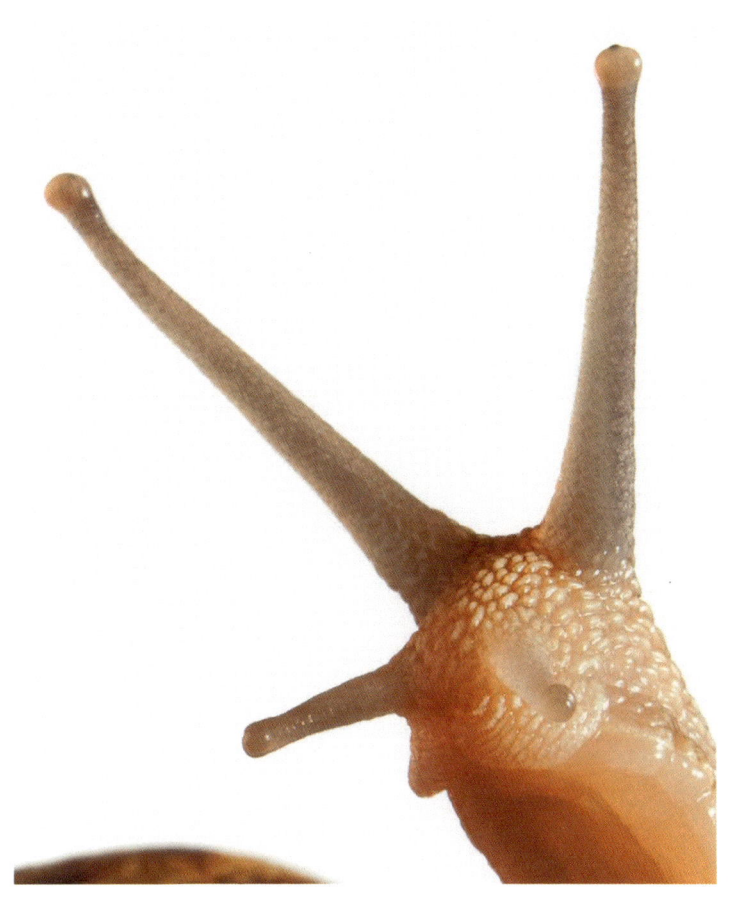

What is this?

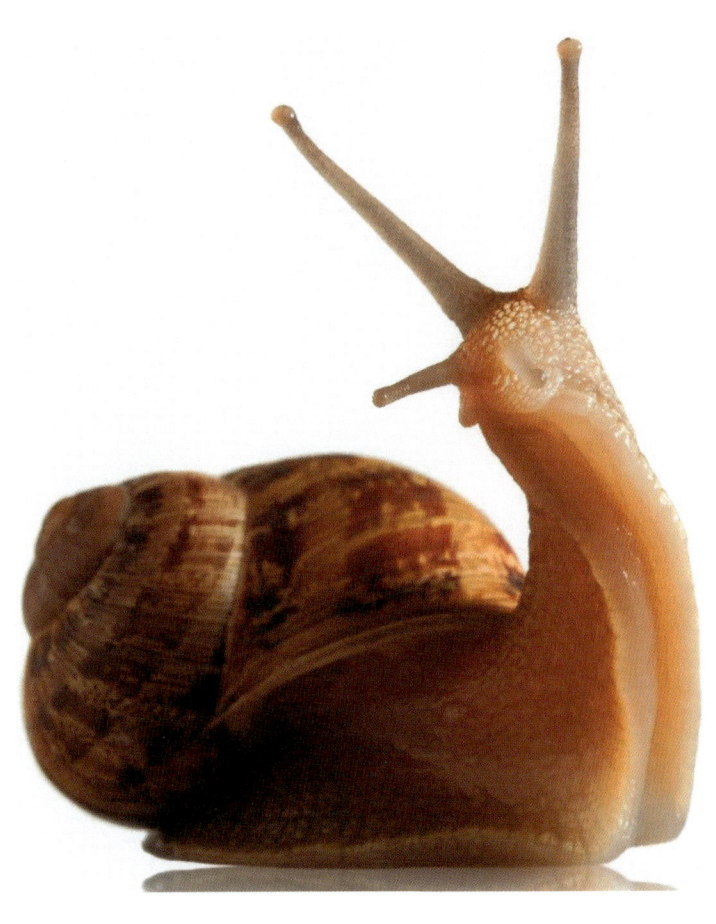

A Snail

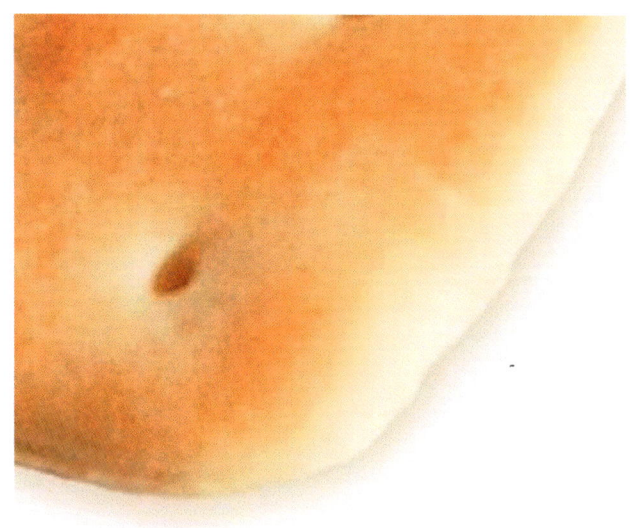

What is this?

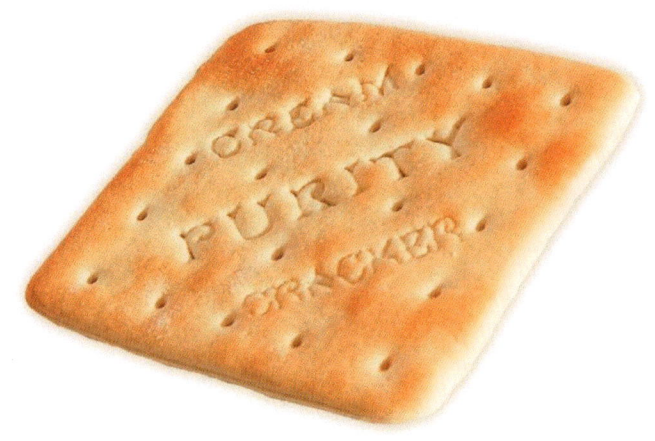

Cream Cracker

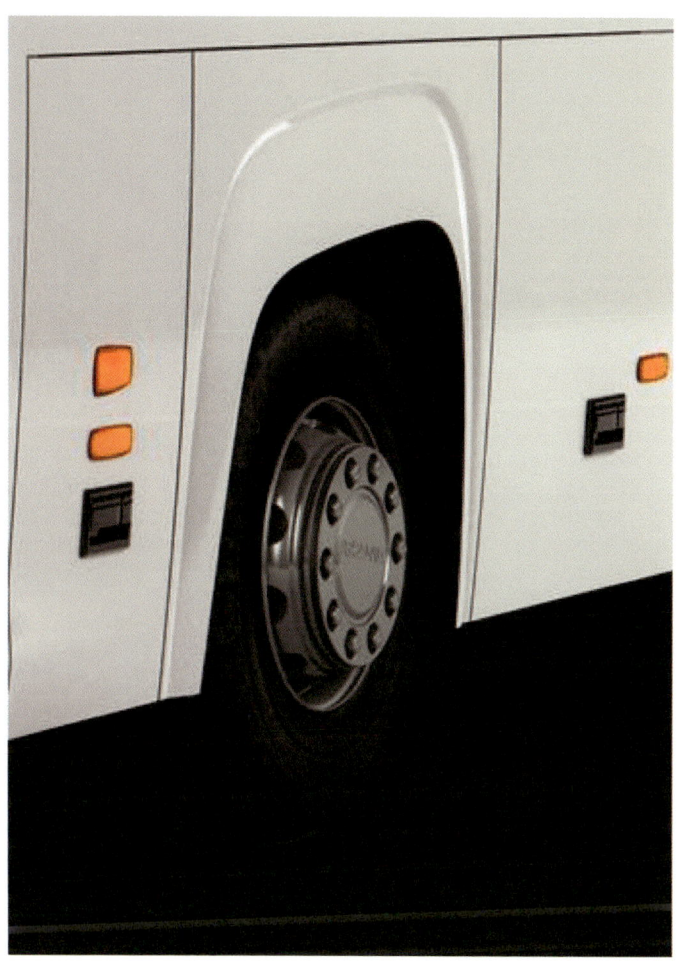

What is this?

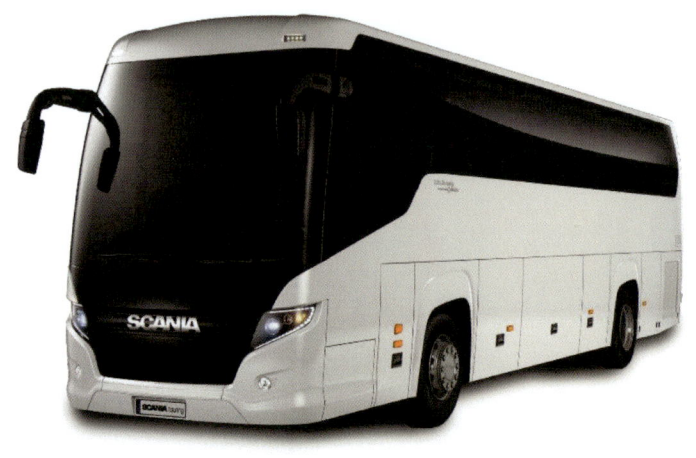

Coach

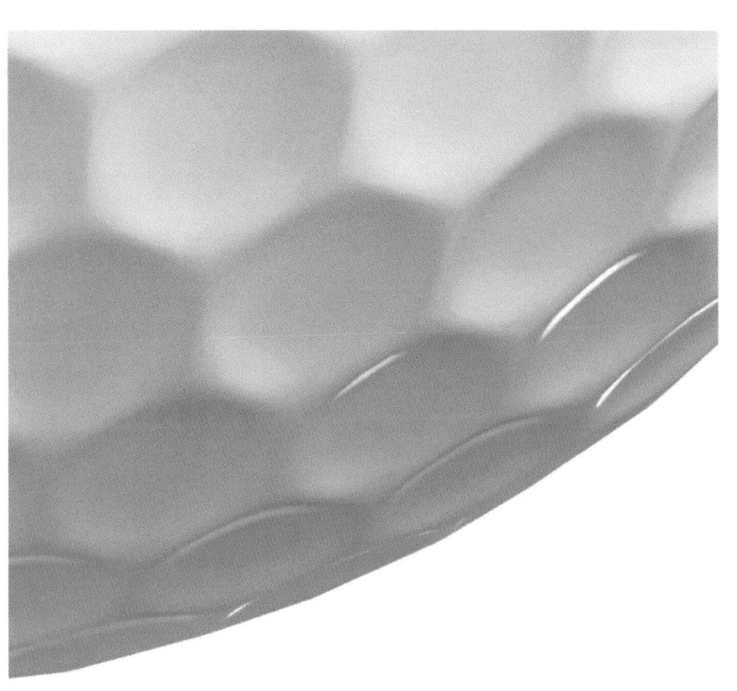

What is this?

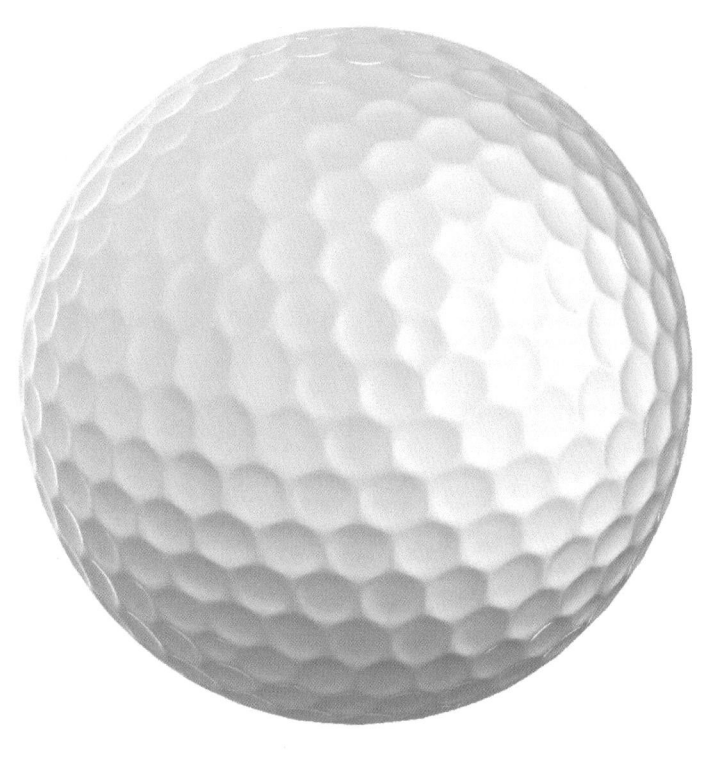

Golf Ball

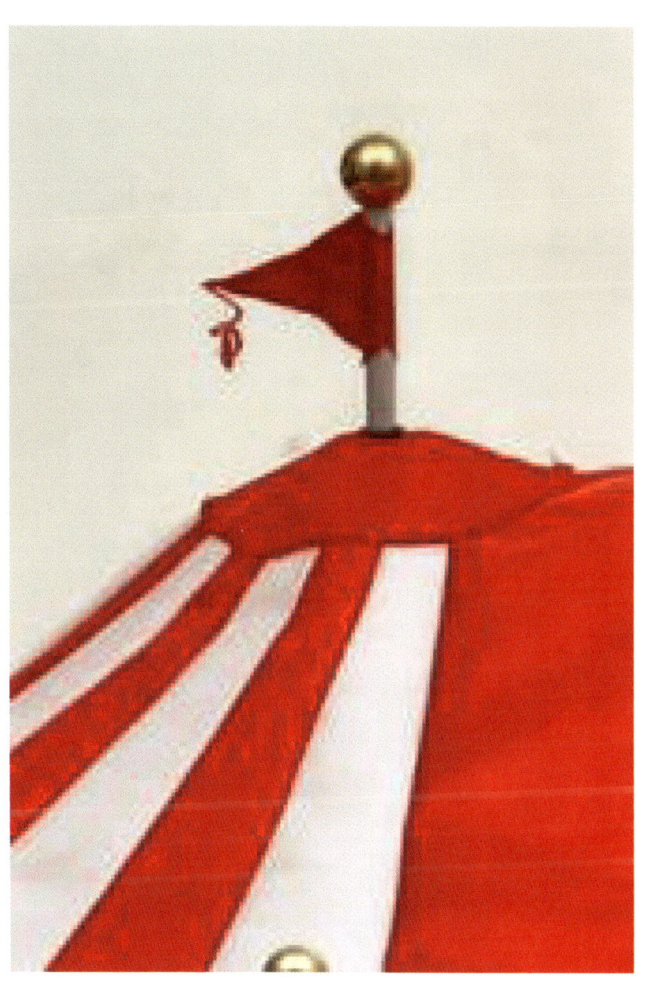

What is this?

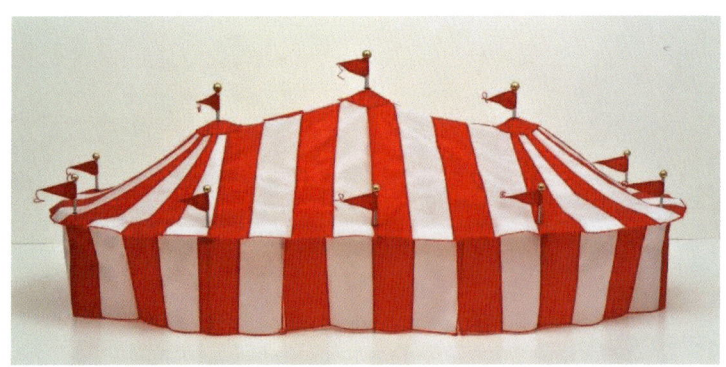

Circus Tent

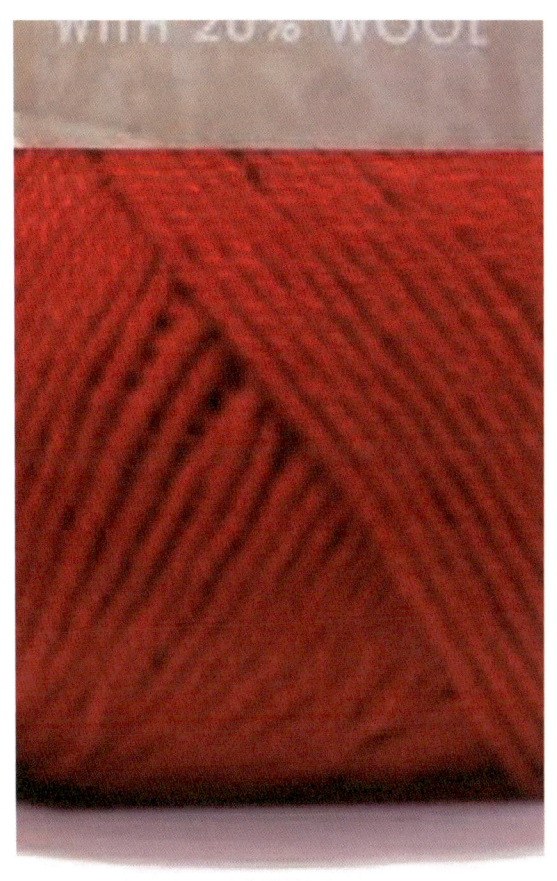

What is this?

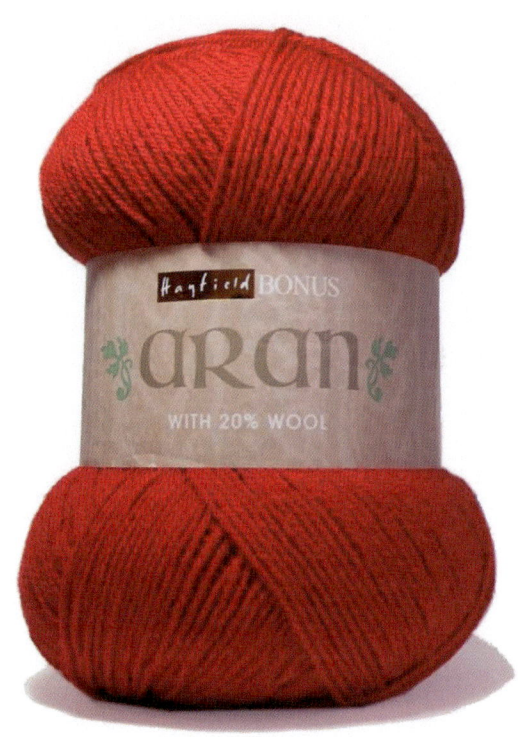

Ball of Wool

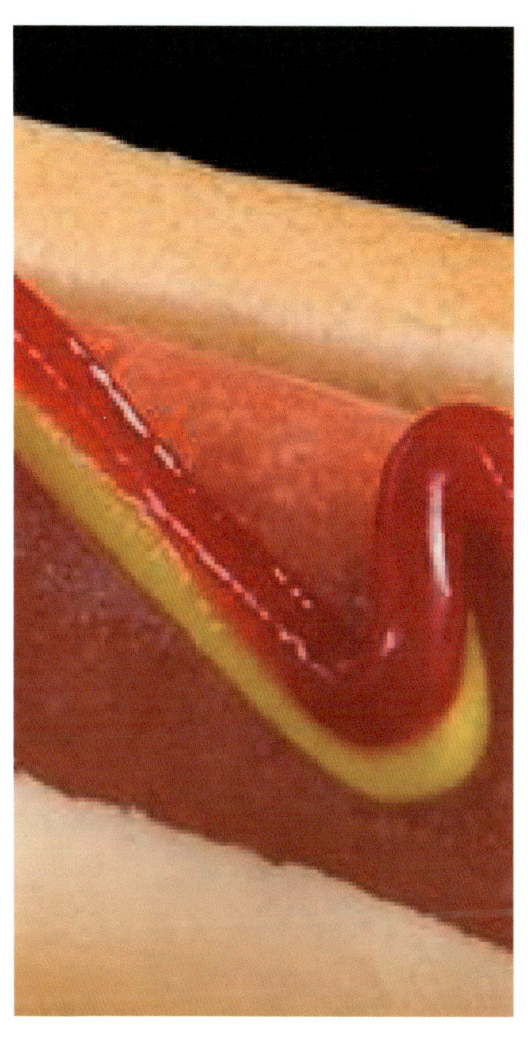

What is this?

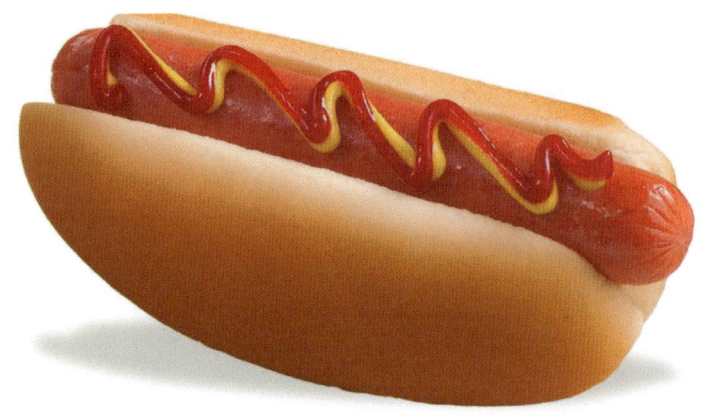

Hot Dog

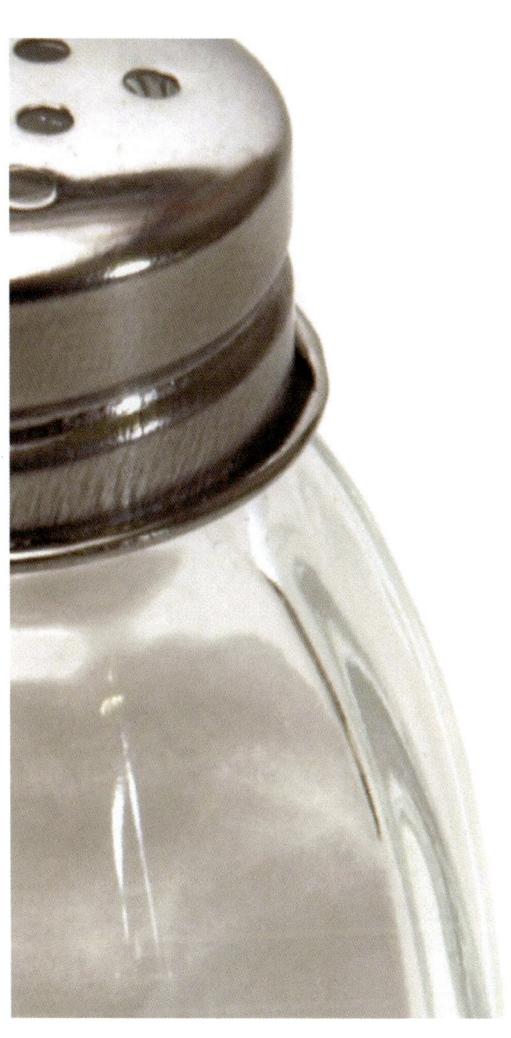

What is this?

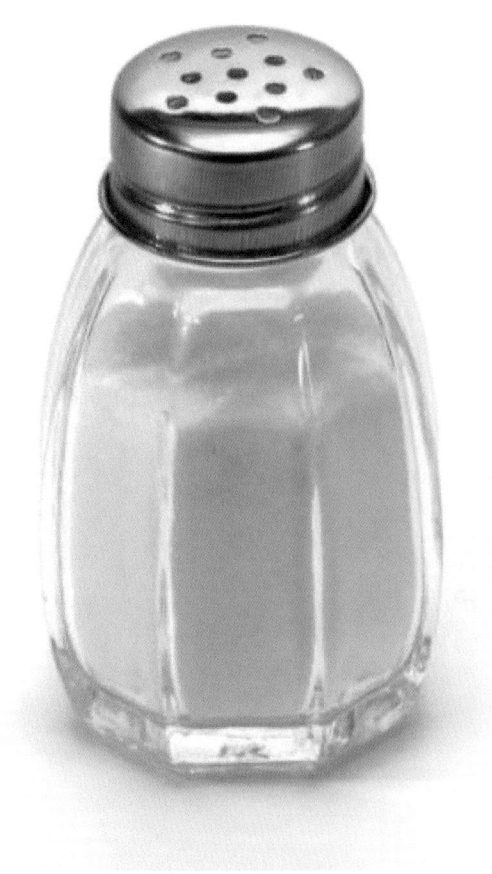

Salt Pot

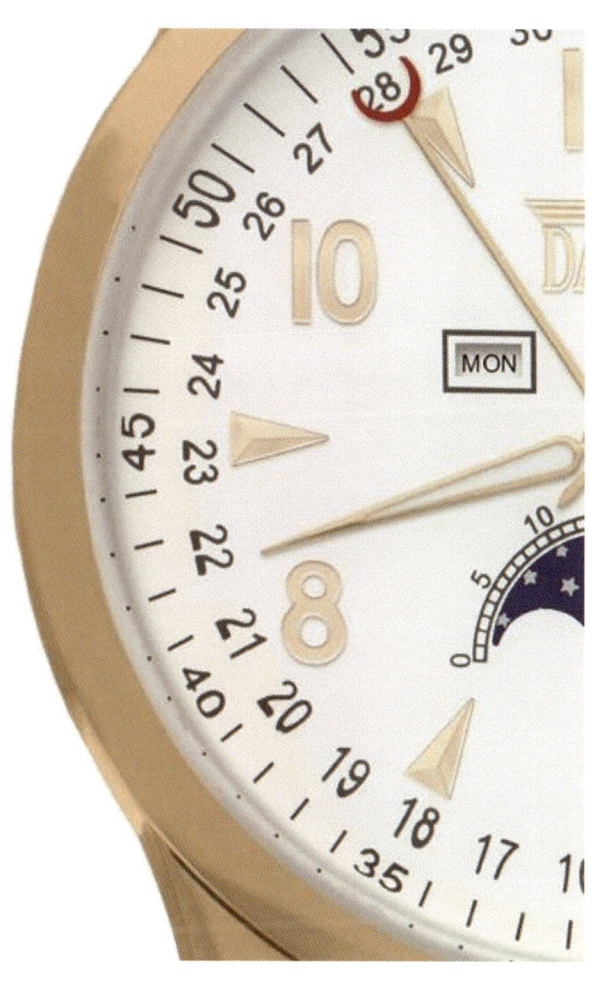

What is this?

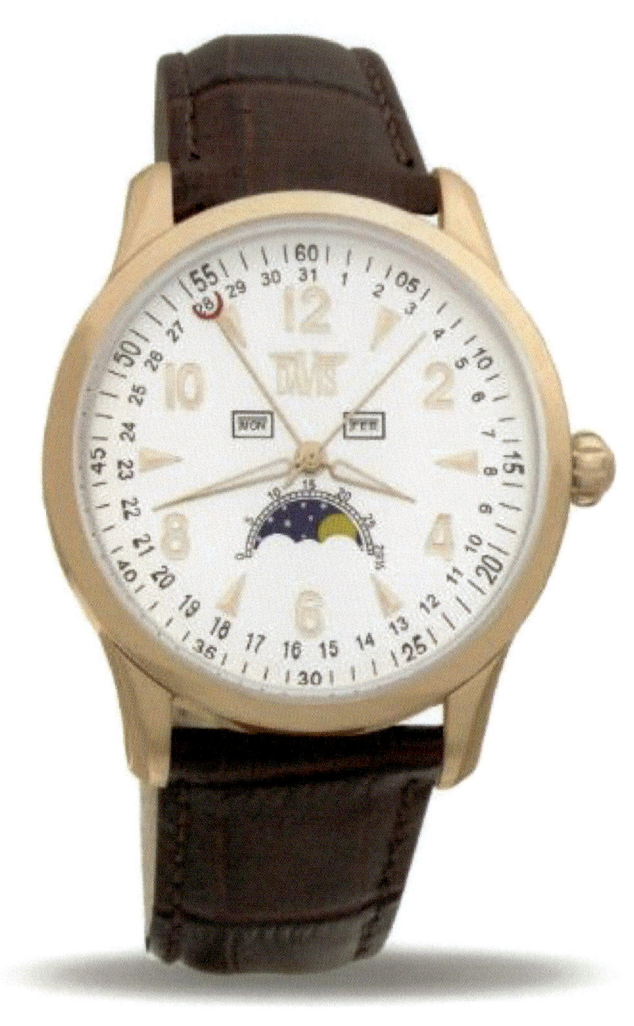

Wrist Watch

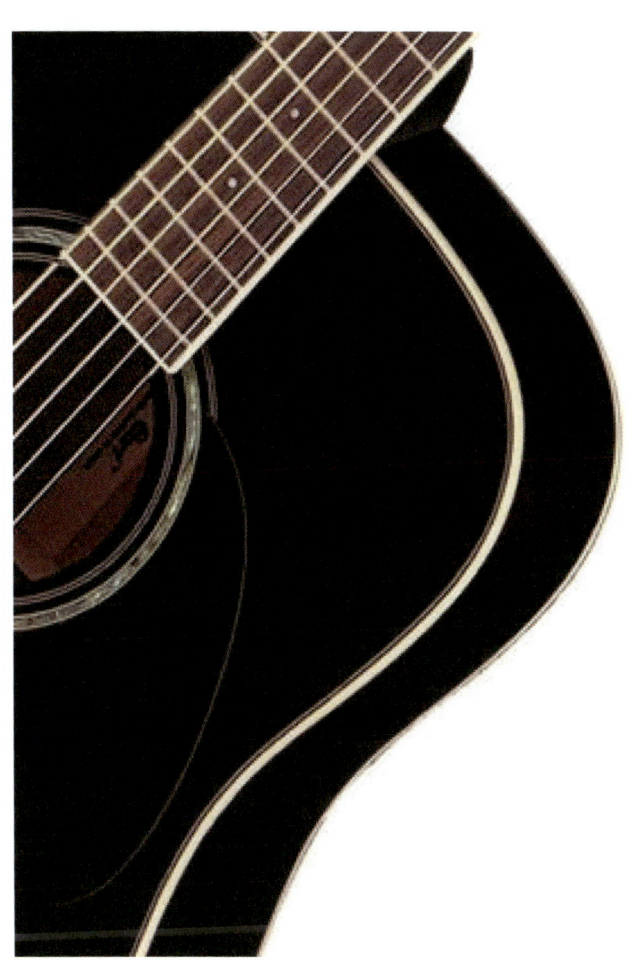

What is this?

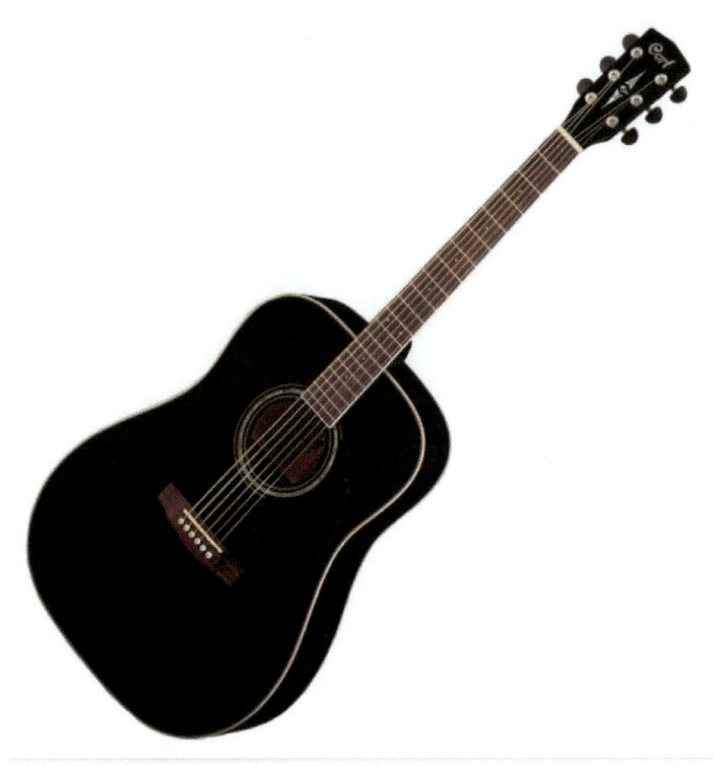

Guitar

Thank you for doing my brain training.

If you liked it, please leave a review on my Amazon Page.

If you didn't like it all feedback is welcome.

Andre Govier

Printed in Great Britain
by Amazon